ANNA CHRISTINA DAUB

Numerical Haemodynamics in the Human Heart

SCHRIFTENREIHE DES INSTITUTS FÜR STRÖMUNGSMECHANIK
KARLSRUHER INSTITUT FÜR TECHNOLOGIE (KIT)

BAND 3

Numerical Haemodynamics in the Human Heart

BY

ANNA CHRISTINA DAUB

KIT Scientific Publishing

Dissertation, Karlsruher Institut für Technologie (KIT)
KIT-Fakultät für Maschinenbau

Tag der mündlichen Prüfung: 11. Januar 2018
Referenten: Prof. Dr.-Ing. B. Frohnapfel
Univ.-Prof. Dr.-Ing. habil. M. Breuer

Impressum

KIT Scientific Publishing

Karlsruher Institut für Technologie (KIT)
KIT Scientific Publishing
Straße am Forum 2
D-76131 Karlsruhe

KIT Scientific Publishing is a registered trademark
of Karlsruhe Institute of Technology.
Reprint using the book cover is not allowed.

www.ksp.kit.edu

Print on Demand 2018 – Gedruckt auf FSC-zertifiziertem Papier

ISSN 2199-8868
ISBN 978-3-7315-0757-4
DOI 10.5445/KSP/1000080044

Abstract

Numerical patient-specific heart models are far from being used in the daily clinical routine: they are complex to generate and generalised post-processing techniques have not been developed yet. The characteristic vortex formation in the ventricles is believed to be affected at an early stage of heart diseases. As such, the identification of flow quantities connected to a patient's health status can yield important insights and help choosing an appropriate minimally invasive treatment. The development of highly simplified models that can be solved with low computational effort and still provide the desired information is therefore the long-term goal scientists strive for. Advancements in this field are the object of the present thesis.

First, post-processing of patient-specific data has to be standardised because meaningful measures are needed in research and clinic. In the present work, the vortex generation is in the focus of the investigation. Combining Eulerian and Lagrangian techniques provides broad information, such as vortex formation and particle residence times. The chosen methods are characterised by means of necessary spatial and temporal resolutions and objective criteria are developed to enable automatic processing of flow data.

Then, valid simplifications for the *in-silico* models have to be identified. Thereby, the goal is to find the best cost-benefit approach. Main target is the mitral valve, as it affects the inflow into the left ventricle. However, its complex motion is challenging and costly to model. Although multiple simplified model options exist, they are rarely validated or compared to one another within the same heart geometry. This work closes one gap by comparing an idealised planar model and a three-dimensional valve in an idealised left ventricle.

Kurzfassung

Numerische patientenspezifische Herzmodelle sind weit davon entfernt im klinischen Alltag angewandt zu werden. Die Erzeugung ist aufwendig und die Nachbearbeitung ist nicht standardisiert. Es wird angenommen, dass die charakteristische Wirbelbildung im Herzen bereits in frühen Krankheitsstadien beeinflusst wird. Strömungsgrößen zu identifizieren, die in Zusammenhang mit dem Gesundheitszustand des Patienten stehen, ist wichtig. Wissenschaftler verfolgen daher als langfristiges Ziel die Entwicklung einfacher Modelle, die schnell gelöst werden können und dennoch wertvolle Informationen liefern. Hierzu liefert diese Arbeit einen Beitrag.

Zunächst muss die Verarbeitung der Daten standardisiert werden, um zuverlässige Maßstäbe in Forschung und Klinik zu generieren. In der vorliegenden Arbeit liegt der Fokus auf der Wirbelidentifikation. Eulersche und Lagrangesche Methoden liefern in Kombination viele Informationen, beispielsweise über Wirbelbildung und Aufenthaltszeiten von Partikeln. Die gewählten Methoden werden im Hinblick auf ihre räumlichen und zeitlichen Auflösungen charakterisiert. Es werden objektive Kriterien entwickelt, die eine automatisierte Verarbeitung der Strömungsdaten ermöglichen.

Anschließend müssen Vereinfachungen der *in-silico* Modelle identifiziert werden. Ziel ist es, die beste Kosten-Nutzen Variante zu finden. Im Fokus liegt die Mitralklappe, da sie die Einströmung in den linken Ventrikel steuert. Allerdings ist die Simulation der komplexen Bewegung schwierig und rechenintensiv. Obwohl verschiedene Modelle existieren, wurden sie selten direkt miteinander verglichen. Die vorliegende Arbeit schließt eine Lücke, indem ein vereinfachtes ebenes Klappenmodell mit einer dreidimensionalen Klappe innerhalb eines vereinfachten Ventrikels verglichen wird.

Table of Contents

1 Introduction

The heart is the organ that keeps the circulatory system running and thus provides the body with all necessary nutrients and oxygen. Nowadays, cardiovascular diseases are still the number one cause of death and responsible for three out of ten deaths throughout the world [112]. If such diseases are recognised early on, many can be treated effectively through proper drug administration or by conducting repairing surgery. However, early diagnosis remains challenging as not all aspects concerning the functioning of the heart are fully understood.

The muscular hollow organ is positioned nearly in the centre of the thorax. It consists of four chambers, two atria and two ventricles, that contract and relax periodically as reaction to the electric stimulation of the sinus node. As seen in Figure 1.1, the muscle is covered by veins and arteries, that provide nutrients necessary for a functioning heart. The large vessels marked with arrows in Figure 1.1 and 1.2, i.e. the superior and inferior vena cava, the pulmonary artery, the pulmonary veins and the aorta, transport the blood from and to the heart. Thereby, de-oxygenated blood travels from the body through the right atrium and ventricle towards the lungs. From the lungs, oxygen-rich blood is guided into the left atrium (LA), from where it is directed into the left ventricle (LV) and pumped into the body. A healthy interventricular septum separates the right and left side of the heart, such that the two blood cycles cannot mix. During each beat, the muscle undergoes a complex twisting deformation. Thereby, the apex, the veins and arteries can be compared to anchors that fix the heart in its position, whereas the pericardium surrounding the heart prevents it from affecting other organs.

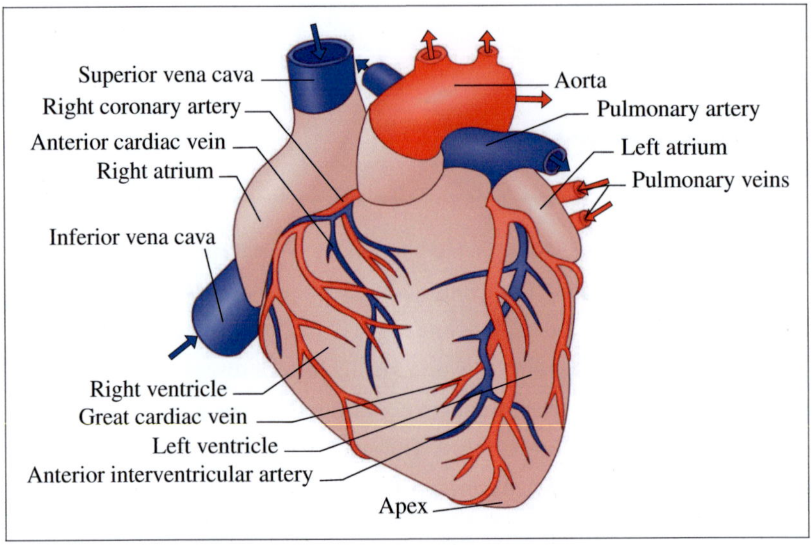

Figure 1.1: The human heart in viewing direction towards a patient. Sketch adapted from Aviva - medical encyclopedia [6].

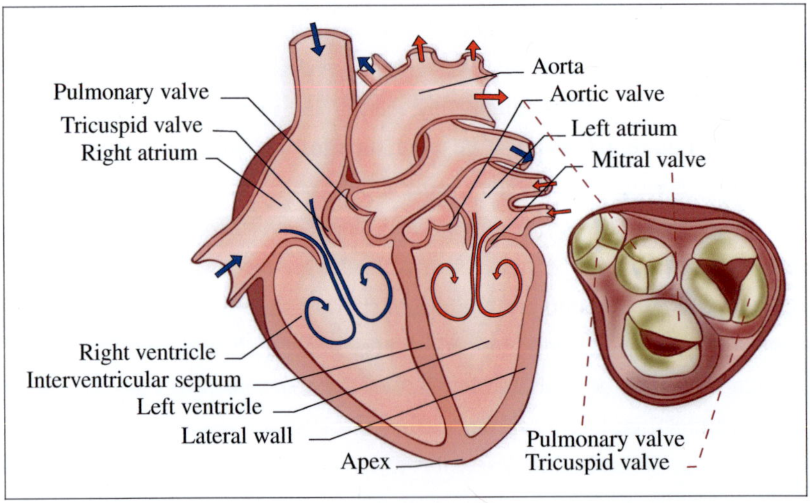

Figure 1.2: (left) The human heart cut in the four chamber view and (right) the four heart valves regarded from the top. Sketch adapted from Aviva - medical encyclopedia [6] and Blausen [10].

Figure 1.2 further illustrates on the right hand side the top view cross-section of the human heart, showing the four heart valves which separate the ventricles from the atria and vessels. It can be seen that the aortic valve, the tricuspid valve and the pulmonary valve have three leaflets, which are in good approximation of the same size and shape and therefore can be modelled in axisymmetric configurations. Out of these three, the aortic valve, which connects the LV with the aorta (compare Figure 1.2, left), is mainly studied in the literature as it determines how the blood enters into the circulatory system. Another reason for conducting studies of the left side of the heart is that the LV has to carry higher loads compared to the right ventricle because it has to pump against a higher resistance imposed by the larger circulatory system.

The heart valve which directly influences the flow characteristics in the LV is the mitral valve (MV). It connects the LA with the LV and consists of only two asymmetrical leaflets. If the opening and closing of the MV develops a dysfunction, the risk of having regurgitation or stenosis rises [1].

1.1 Motivation

Conventional indices used for the characterisation of cardiac performance, such as the ejection fraction (EF), usually do not reveal significant changes until there is an overt heart dysfunction. As such, these indices are less effective for the early diagnosis and treatment of cardiac diseases. In the last decades, the blood flow in the human heart has been studied intensively and it was found that the blood dynamics are immediately affected by changes in the cardiac function [84]. Consequently, understanding the flow dynamics can enhance the overall understanding of the cardiovascular system and thus help to identify cardiovascular disorders and to plan a proper minimal invasive treatment [11]. Studying the haemodynamics directly on the patient is not impossible yet inefficient. For instance, a color-Doppler echo-cardiogram can deliver highly time-resolved two-dimensional (2D) velocity data but the important third velocity component is missing. Three-dimensional (3D) phase contrast cardiovascular magnetic resonance can cope with this problem but is not yet able to provide the desired temporal resolution. Further, all kinds of measurement techniques directly employed at the patient are not able to forecast any surgical outcomes. In order to fully understand the heart flow characteristics, it is necessary to develop computational heart models that provide the desired insights.

Today's computational techniques and resources enable the study of patient-specific blood flow in *in-silico* models. Unfortunately, the models are far from being used in clinical application as they are highly complex and many intermediate steps are necessary before reliable patient-specific conclusions can be drawn. If a proper model is extracted into a numerical setup, the conduction of the calculation needs appropriate resources, which is usually expensive in terms of computational resources as well as computational time. Therefore, the long-term goal has to be the development of highly simplified models that can be solved with low computational effort and still provide the desired information.

McQueen and Peskin [74] have laid the foundation of numerical heart models by choosing the heart as application example for the implementation of the immersed boundary method. They started by immersing a toroidal, fibre-wound tube into a viscous, incompressible fluid and step-wise extended their model to cover the whole heart with its two atria and ventricles, including gross captures of the heart valves [59].

The valves allow blood to flow in one defined direction and prevent the backward flow of the blood. Thus, they have a non-negligible influence on the flow characteristics found in the heart. A heart valve consists of soft tissue that undergoes large deformations and highly interacts with the surrounding blood. Modelling this kind of fluid-structure interaction is still challenging. This explains why most available computational heart models include simplified valve models that are supposed to mimic the valves' behaviour. However, the different available models are rarely validated or compared to one another within the same heart geometry.

Solely Kunzelman et al. [50] present a physiological 3D mitral valve simulated in the framework of fluid-structure interaction. However, the geometry is not implemented into a ventricle but into a simplified computational box. Other attempts to include fluid-structure interaction are found in 2D within ventricles of varying complexity [1, 17, 24, 94]. Most research teams work with simplified valve models. For example, Bavo et al. [8] present a 3D valve geometry whose motion is prescribed. They recommend the usage of 3D valves in heart flow simulations, as the leaflets highly influence the ventricular flow field. Seo et al. [86] agree with these findings and show that a highly simplified valve by means of a simple opening and closing of the valve plane does not yield physiological flow characteristics. However, other groups, e.g. Saber et al. [77] or Vedula et al. [102], obtain promising results with the same simple valve model. Further refinement of this simplest approach yields a step-wise opening and closing of the valve plane which still does not involve 3D valves. Thereby, the effective opening area of the valve shall be mimicked. Results presented by different research groups show good agreement with the expected flow characteristics [7, 67, 68, 80].

If the heart is healthy, its inflow characteristics are dominated by a ring shaped vortex that forms behind the MV and then propagates towards the apex. Thereby, the LV is washed out, risks of flow stasis and thrombosis are minimised and a smooth transition from filling to ejection is supported. In this respect, the requirements of post-processing strategies centre around the necessity to accurately determine and characterise the vortices. Numerous post-processing tools aiming at fulfilling this task are available. However, there is currently no standardised strategy for analysing and visualising the blood flow in the human heart which is essential for meaningful and reliable comparison of data generated with different setups, e.g. comparing simulations with different MV models.

Based on point-wise Eulerian calculations, local vortex detection methods like the Q-criterion provide the majority of the desired information on the spatio-temporal development of the vortex formation process. However, cause-effect relations between inflow properties, shape of the heart wall and vortex formation remain hidden, since only instantaneous velocity fields are evaluated consecutively. Performing additional Lagrangian analysis by means of the finite-time Lyapunov exponent accounts for this issue. Its capability to visualise the transport of Lagrangian coherent structures enables the identification of clear vortex boundaries and recirculation zones. Furthermore, the finite-time Lyapunov exponent captures the time-dependent evolution of the dynamic system [88].

Both introduced post-processing methods are well accepted and widely used for researching blood flow in the human heart. As full characterisation and guidelines for consistent application – especially for the finite-time Lyapunov exponent – are missing, a systematic variation of the spatial and temporal resolution is necessary. A fully generalised post-processing procedure enables reliable and meaningful comparison of flow changes introduced in the LV by geometrical changes, e.g. remodelling after a heart attack, or changing health status, e.g. dysfunction of the MV.

1.2 Objectives and Procedure

The objective of this thesis is the identification of valid simplifications for the scope of application in computational heart models in comparison to the physiological human heart. To achieve this goal, two major steps are necessary. Firstly, it is important to ensure a trustworthy post-processing that allows the extraction of meaningful data. Secondly, the role of the MV model in terms of vortex generation in the LV has to be investigated and described.

Therefore, the physiological flow characteristics in the heart, the conservation equations describing the flow problem and the available options of describing wall movement numerically are demonstrated in the first place.

Against this backdrop, the applied post-processing techniques, namely the Q-criterion and the finite-time Lyapunov exponent, are examined on test cases in order to ensure a reliable judgement of the simulation results. Thereby, a step towards generalisation is taken by analysing the spatial and temporal resolution of the underlying Eulerian velocity data. Additionally, the spatial resolution of the Lagrangian particle tracking is varied to complete the characterisation of the finite-time Lyapunov exponent. This procedure enables the derivation of global criteria to estimate the required data resolution.

Prior to examining heart flow results, some simplifications commonly used in modelling biomechanics are discussed. Hereby, the non-Newtonian properties of blood flow, possible transition from laminar to turbulent flow and geometrical simplifications resulting from image processing is included. These considerations build the basis for the conducted simulations.

For a complete overview, the available MV model types are reviewed before the most promising ones are implemented into an idealised model of the LA and the LV. Based on the simulation results, the influence of the MV models on the flow characteristics is discussed. The main focus lies on the impact of the respective MV model on the accuracy of the obtained result, namely the vortex dynamics in the LV. Herein, the possibility to trim low cost models to mimic the physiological flow in the LV is evaluated.

Finally, the identified valid simplifications are implemented into a patient-specific LV, in order to demonstrate their applicability under physiological conditions. Recapitulating the obtained results allows to draw conclusions which lead to suggestions for following projects.

2 Fundamentals

The physiological blood flow in the human heart is dominated by a vortex formation process which is described first in this chapter. An appropriate numerical description of such complex flow must include these flow dynamics. The governing equations that need to be solved numerically are introduced including first simplifications. A major challenge in transferring a physiological heart into an *in-silico* model is the description of the moving heart walls and valve leaflets. Therefore, different possibilities of incorporating wall movement in numerical models are presented and discussed in the last section.

2.1 Flow Characteristics in the Human Heart

The heart is a muscular organ that pumps four to five litres of blood per minute through the circulatory system by periodically contracting and relaxing. The four valves regulate the blood flow with their flexible leaflets, which open only unidirectionally. Besides the MV, which is the only valve with two asymmetric leaflets, the heart valves have three nearly uniform leaflets.

The pressure difference at the two sides of a valve drives its opening and closure. It is the reason for which a heart cycle is typically drawn in a pressure-volume diagram (compare Figure 2.1). During the early diastolic phase, the isochoric relaxation, the pressure in the ventricles drops under the pressure in the atria and thus causes the MV and the tricuspid valve to open. The filling phase follows and is accompanied by a slight pressure increase towards the end of the diastole. The systolic phase starts with an isochoric contraction that causes the two open valves to close and lasts until the pressure in the right ventricle and the LV overcomes the pressure in the aorta and the pulmonary artery. With the opening of the aortic and pulmonary valve, the second part of the systole – the ejection phase – begins. Meanwhile, the pressure in the ventricles decreases again and drops below the pressure in the aorta and the pulmonary artery. As a consequence, the aortic valve and the pulmonary valve are forced to close and the cycle starts over with the isochoric relaxation.

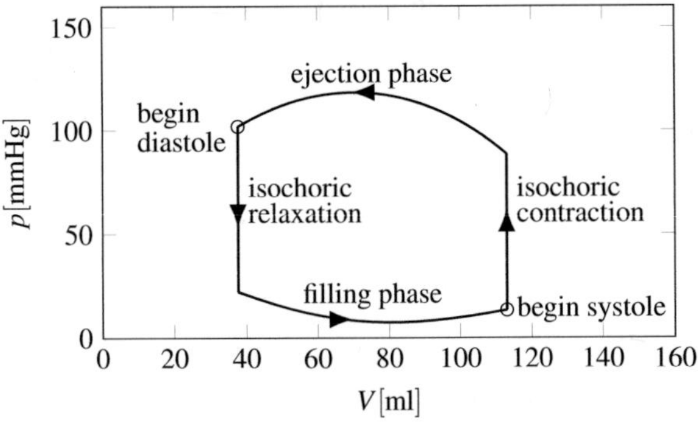

Figure 2.1: Sketch of a typical pressure-volume diagram in the ventricle for one heart beat. Sketch adapted from Spiegel [92].

At the beginning of the filling process, an intake jet enters into each of the two ventricles. These jets are accompanied by the formation of a vortex ring occurring at about one quarter of a cardiac cycle. It is induced by the rolling up of the shear layer that develops at the leaflet tips between the nearly resting fluid in the ventricle and the impinging jet. The resulting velocity gradients promote a vorticity flux from the surrounding fluid into the vortex ring. Therefore, the vortex grows and balances out the deceleration of the intake jet into the ventricular fluid nearly at rest. As the diastole continues, the motion of the cardiac myocardium causes the vortex ring to further increase in size while its velocity decreases. There is no flow through the apex of the ventricle at this time. As the intake process continues further, the vortex interacts with the lateral heart wall and inclines towards the apex of the ventricle. At this point the velocity of the intake jet decreases until the filling is completed and the MV closes. Impinging at the apex and without the jet feeding inertia into the flow, the vortex rapidly becomes unstable and breaks down into smaller structures.

The expulsion phase begins with the opening of the aortic valve. First, the vortex in the aortic channel, a remain of the previous heart beat, is rinsed out. Then, the blood is directed towards the aorta in a helical motion. At the end of the systole the vortex structures in the left and right ventricles have nearly vanished and only a small vortex in front of the outlet valves remains.

2.2 Governing Equations of Fluid Dynamics

In this section the formulation of the governing conservation equations is given and some simplifications are discussed. A more detailed description with additional derivations can for example be found in [82].

The motion of fluids in general is described by a set of conservation equations, which are valid as long as the fluid within the volume of interest can be described as a continuum – a hypothetically continuous matter. In the present work, blood is treated on the macroscopic level and thus represented as a homogeneous suspension of blood plasma and cellular components. This assumption only holds true for large arteries and vessels where no separation of liquid and cells is observed. The required conservation equations consist of conservation of mass, also known as the continuity equation, and conservation of momentum. The conservation of energy is neglected, as the temperature is considered to be constant through the region of interest.

The conservation of mass and momentum are given in index notation for a Cartesian coordinate system as

$$\frac{\partial \rho}{\partial t} + \frac{\partial(\rho u_i)}{\partial x_i} = 0, \tag{2.1}$$

$$\rho\left(\frac{\partial u_i}{\partial t} + u_j \frac{\partial u_i}{\partial x_j}\right) = -\frac{\partial p}{\partial x_i} + \frac{\partial \tau_{ij}}{\partial x_j} + \rho f_i. \tag{2.2}$$

Here, the vector of velocity is given by $u_i = (u_1, u_2, u_3)$ in the three coordinate directions, $x_i = (x_1, x_2, x_3)$. Further, pressure is denoted by p, f_i are the externally acting volume forces and ρ is the fluid density. For incompressible fluids, the continuity equation reduces to

$$\frac{\partial u_i}{\partial x_i} = 0. \tag{2.3}$$

The stress tensor, τ_{ij}, contains the viscous stresses exerted on the fluid. As the stress tensor consists of six unknown independent components, the system of four equations needs to be closed in order to obtain a solution. This is done by incorporating a constitutive equation which connects the dynamic fluid viscosity, μ, with the exhibited stresses. In the case of treating blood flow as homogeneous suspension with an effective viscosity μ_{eff}, the constitutive equation for Newtonian fluid,

$$\tau_{ij} = \mu_{eff}\left(\frac{\partial u_i}{\partial x_j} + \frac{\partial u_j}{\partial x_i}\right) - \frac{2}{3}\mu_{eff}\frac{\partial u_k}{\partial x_k}, \tag{2.4}$$

can be used. The last term in Equation (2.4) is equal to zero due to continuity. Blood is known to have a compressibility of $3.75 \cdot 10^{-10}\,\frac{\mathrm{m}^2}{\mathrm{N}}$ [108], which yields that the pressure changes in the heart result in density changes of approximately $5 \cdot 10^{-4}\%$. This effect is considered negligible and thus blood can be treated as incompressible, as is done in the present work. However, introducing a slight compressibility into the numerical solver can have stabilising effects on the solution procedure [104].

Together with the assumptions of incompressibility and isothermal behaviour, the small height differences throughout the domain in comparison to the whole circulatory system yields that no buoyancy effects occur. Thus, the acceleration due to gravity is neglected. $f_i = 0$ holds true, because gravity is the only acceleration in question to contribute to the volume forces.

Inserting the introduced simplifications, the so called Navier-Stokes equations (NSE) result from the momentum equations

$$\rho\left(\frac{\partial u_i}{\partial t}+u_j\frac{\partial u_i}{\partial x_j}\right)=-\frac{\partial p}{\partial x_i}+\mu_{eff}\left(\frac{\partial^2 u_i}{\partial x_j \partial x_j}\right). \tag{2.5}$$

Equation (2.3) and (2.5) form a system of equations, which fully describes the motion of blood flow in the heart and large arteries.

It is demonstrated in the following that the transformation of the NSE (2.5) into their dimensionless form yields the definition of important dimensionless indicators. For this purpose, the dimensional flow variables are scaled by corresponding characteristic quantities. The resulting dimensionless quantities are marked with *, such that

$$u_i^\star=\frac{u_i}{U_c};\quad x_i^\star=\frac{x_i}{L_c};\quad t^\star=t\omega;\quad p^\star=\frac{p}{\rho U_c^2}, \tag{2.6}$$

where U_c, L_c and ω are the characteristic velocity, length scale and angular frequency. Replacing the dimensional quantities with their dimensionless counterpart, the system of Equations (2.3) and (2.5) can now be written in a dimensionless form, as

$$\frac{\partial u_i^\star}{\partial x_i^\star}=0, \tag{2.7}$$

$$\frac{\mathrm{Wo}^2}{\mathrm{Re}}\frac{\partial u_i^\star}{\partial t^\star}+u_j^\star\frac{\partial u_i^\star}{\partial x_j^\star}=-\frac{\partial p^\star}{\partial x_i^\star}+\frac{1}{\mathrm{Re}}\left(\frac{\partial^2 u_i^\star}{\partial x_j^\star \partial x_j^\star}\right). \tag{2.8}$$

In the non-dimensional equations, two dimensionless numbers appear: the Reynolds number, Re, and the Womersley number, Wo, defined as

$$\mathrm{Re}=\frac{\rho U_c L_c}{\mu_{eff}};\qquad \mathrm{Wo}=L_c\sqrt{\frac{\rho\omega}{\mu_{eff}}}. \tag{2.9}$$

The Reynolds number is the most important indicator used in fluid mechanics. It relates the inertial forces to the viscous forces in the flow. For the human heart the characteristic length is usually chosen equal to the hydraulic diameter of the heart valve open during the respective phase. Thereby, the Reynolds number in a healthy human left ventricle reaches $\mathrm{Re} \approx 3000-4000$ at peak systole [72]. During the diastole the Reynolds number is typically below the systolic range [69] due to a smaller peak velocity.

The Womersley number is used to characterise periodic flows. It relates the transient inertial forces to the shear forces, such that it allows conclusions on the shape of the velocity profile and on the phase shift between the bulk velocity and the driving pressure gradient. In a pulsating pipe flow, if $\mathrm{Wo} \ll 1$, the velocity profile is parabolic and in phase with the pressure gradient, whereas if $\mathrm{Wo} \gg 1$, the velocity profile is flat and the bulk velocity reacts in a 90° phase shift to the driving pressure gradient [101]. In the human heart, the Womersley number varies between 20 and 30 [69]. Combination of Re and Wo,

$$\mathrm{St} = \frac{\mathrm{Wo}^2}{2\pi\mathrm{Re}} = \frac{L_c}{U_c T_c}, \tag{2.10}$$

results in the Strouhal number, St. Small Strouhal numbers ($\mathrm{St} \leq 0.05$) determined for the heart flow can be an indicator of heart diseases [21] and thus should be determined when a patient-specific flow is analysed.

2.3 Numerical Reproduction of Moving Walls

Physiological simulation of the blood flow through the human heart involves the necessity of numerically reproducing the heart wall movement which drives the flow. Additionally, it might be necessary to describe the movement of valve leaflets through the fluid domain. Besides simpler strategies, e.g. the definition of sink and source terms over the heart wall mimicking the wall movement as reported by Alkemper (2017) or Vellguth (2017), two major approaches which fully resolve the wall motion are available, namely prescription of the wall movement or fluid-structure interaction (FSI). The first, prescription of the wall movement, only determines the reaction of the flow to the moving boundary. Elasticity effects or changing pressure distribution do not affect the domain boundary. The second, FSI, includes solving a structural domain that reacts to changing flow conditions. Thus, a prescription of wall movement is easier to realise, but information on the wall movement needs to be known a priori and strains or stresses within the structure remain unknown.

All simulations are carried out using the open source software OpenFOAM (Open Source Field Operation and Manipulation). The two releases used, namely OpenFOAM-1.6-ext and foam-extend 3.1, are highlighted throughout the following chapters whenever relevant. In general, the capability of including wall movement is already available. The specific case implemented within the framework of this thesis is introduced in Chapter 3.3.

Disregarding the choice between prescribed motion or FSI, the spatial discretisation of the fluid domain (fluid mesh) can be treated either in an arbitrary Lagrangian-Eulerian (ALE) description, where the mesh adapts to the moving boundary, or in a pure Eulerian formulation, where the moving wall is immersed into the fluid mesh by means of the immersed boundary method (IBM). Both formulations are presented in the following. Additionally, an introduction to the treatment of FSI problems is given.

2.3.1 Arbitrary Lagrangian Eulerian Description

As the name already suggests, the ALE formulation combines the Lagrangian and Eulerian formulation in fluid mechanics [100]. Typically, the NSE (2.5) are formulated in an Eulerian framework, where the centre of the analysis is a control volume fixed in space and the behaviour of the fluid passing through the observed control volume as time passes is described. In a pure Eulerian framework the mesh is not moving. A solver determines the change over time of field variables at a specific location. In the Lagrangian formulation, the volume of interest consists of a specific fluid volume and the observer moves with this volume. As such, it describes the change of the initial state including deformation. A pure Lagrangian formulation requires a mesh that moves with the fluid. The mixture of these two points of view results in a moving mesh whose movement is determined by the movement of the computational domain boundary but independent of the internal fluid movement.

The mesh motion has to be solved in an additional set of differential equations. Thereby, the necessary boundary conditions are the prescribed wall movement in the three coordinate directions. OpenFOAM uses a Laplace equation

$$\frac{\partial}{\partial x_j}\left(k\frac{\partial u_i}{\partial x_j}\right) = 0, \tag{2.11}$$

where the mesh diffusivity k is dependent on the distance between the current mesh cell centre and the moving boundary face. This dependency can be chosen to be linear, quadratic or exponential. Figure 2.2 shows an ALE mesh inside a simplified 2D LV with the internal fluid volume, Ω_f, at peak systole and the resultant deformed mesh at peak diastole using a prescribed movement of the boundary, Γ, and a distance-based quadratic diffusivity for calculation of the mesh motion.

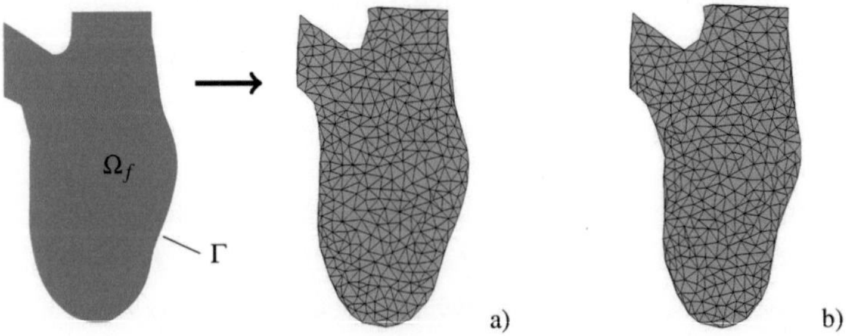

Figure 2.2: Body conformal mesh in an idealised LV at a) peak diastole and b) peak systole.

In the NSE (2.5), the mesh movement is taken into account by replacing the velocity, u_i, in the convective terms with the velocity relative to the mesh motion velocity, c_i, such that

$$\rho\left(\frac{\partial u_i}{\partial t}+u_j\frac{\partial(u_i-c_i)}{\partial x_j}\right)=-\frac{\partial p}{\partial x_i}+\mu_{eff}\left(\frac{\partial^2 u_i}{\partial x_j\partial x_j}\right). \tag{2.12}$$

Herein, the mesh motion velocity, c_i, has to satisfy the space conservation law which relates the rate of change of a control volume to the velocity of its surface [12, 20, 25] by

$$\frac{\mathrm{d}}{\mathrm{d}t}\iiint_V \mathrm{d}V-\iint_S c_i n_i \mathrm{d}S=0. \tag{2.13}$$

Other approximation techniques may lead to errors in the mass conservation that accumulate with time. In case of an incompressible fluid, the cell volume change is equal to the divergence of the mesh velocity, such that the continuity equation (2.1) remains unaffected [25]. In OpenFOAM a second-order discretisation based on three time levels is applied for solving Equation (2.13) [44]. Thereby, the change of the cell volumes is explicitly computed based on the grid node motion (compare Equation (2.11)).

In terms of wall movement, the ALE formulation has the advantage of direct application of the no slip boundary condition. At the wall, u_i has to be equal to c_i, which can be directly imposed, resulting in a Dirichlet boundary condition. In general, standard boundary conditions can be applied without restrictions, e.g. the Dirichlet condition, where the value of a variable is given, and the Neumann condition, where the variable gradient in the wall normal direction is given. Thereby, the set of governing equations yields a pure Lagrangian configuration directly at the wall where the mesh moves with the fluid. The further away from the wall, the more the equations approximate the Eulerian formulation. The generated meshes have boundaries that can reproduce the boundary of the fluid domain exactly and are called body conformal. Thereby, the accuracy of the results at the wall depend on the chosen discretisation and solvers. At the same time the generation of a body conformal mesh within a complex geometry can be challenging. Another disadvantage of the usage of the ALE formulation is the restriction to small movements as highly skewed cells introduce large errors in the results. To solve this problem, remeshing during the simulation process might become necessary. This procedure involves the interpolation of previously determined flow fields onto the new mesh. Both, the interpolation and the mesh generation, produce extra computational costs that depend on the chosen methods.

Regarding the heart flow simulations, the ALE formulation is very attractive as long as the heart valves and the physiological surface of the ventricular wall shall not be fully resolved. Considering only the movement of a smooth ventricular wall, the mesh motion remains manageable without the necessity of remeshing. However, if a physiological rough wall surface is to be considered, a mesh with appropriate resolution to study the effect of the roughness results in million of cells. Additionally, the pre-processing of meshing is challenging, which makes the clinical applicability unrealistic. The description of the heart valves entail another challenge in addition to their large movements. A complete closure of the valves results in cells of zero volume. Special treatment of this scenario includes remeshing and changing mesh topology [8, 15] or strategies of incomplete valve closure [8, 86, 115].

2.3.2 Immersed Boundary Method

The IBM is a non-body conformal method, where the geometry is immersed as surface mesh into a Cartesian volume mesh. Figure 2.3 shows that the mesh itself is then not affected by the movement of the geometry. Thereby, no computational effort is invested into mesh motion and the immersed geometry can be of high complexity and incorporate large deformations without the necessity of remeshing.

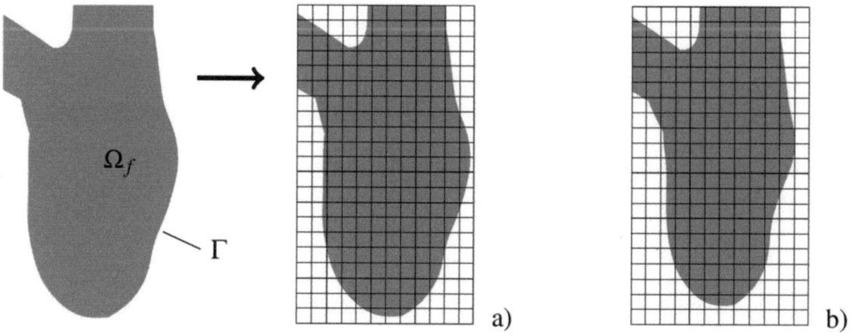

Figure 2.3: Non-body conformal mesh in an idealised LV at a) peak diastole and b) peak systole.

As consequence of the non-body conformal mesh, the boundary condition of a moving wall cannot be directly transferred. Instead, it is incorporated via modification of the governing equations. In general, a source term or forcing function is added into the equations [61], which aims at the reproduction of a boundary condition used in ALE formulation. A forcing function can be included in two different ways. It is either included into the continuous set of equations prior to discretisation, called continuous forcing approach, or it is added to the discretised equations, called discrete forcing approach. Overall, the latter method is more robust in terms of stability and better replicates the shape of the immersed boundary (IB). Further, it is generally applicable once a solver is set up, while the continuous forcing approach has to be reformulated in dependency of the immersed geometry. The continuous forcing approach is not used in the present thesis and the reader is referred to [61] for further information.

The IBM is available for OpenFOAM-1.6-ext in form of a supplemental toolkit which is not distributed with the official release. The implementation is based on a discrete forcing approach. As shown in Figure 2.4, the mesh is divided by the immersed surface, Γ, into a fluid area, Ω_f (dark grey) and a solid area, Ω_s (white). All cells whose centre point is located in the solid region are marked as solid. No flow quantities are stored or solved within those cells. Along the solid surface, Γ, a layer of IB cells (light grey) separates the fluid and the solid part. The IB cells are cut by the immersed surface and their centre point lies in the fluid region. Thus, the flow quantities have to be determined for these cells. The basic idea is that the values in the IB cells are interpolated based on the neighbouring fluid and IB cells so as to fulfil the Dirichlet boundary condition at the immersed surface. More specifically, a quadratic polynomial is used to determine the value of a variable, Φ, in the cell centre point, P, as

$$\begin{aligned}\Phi_P =&\Phi_{IB} + C_0(x_P - x_{IB}) + C_1(y_P - y_{IB})\\ &+ C_2(x_P - x_{IB})(y_P - y_{IB}) + C_3(x_P - x_{IB})^2 + C_4(y_P - y_{IB})^2.\end{aligned} \tag{2.14}$$

Here, Φ_{IB} denotes the value of variable Φ on the immersed surface and the constants C_0 to C_4 are determined via a weighted least squares method using the extended stencil cross-hatched in Figure 2.4. If a Neumann boundary condition is to be employed at P, a local coordinate system (x', y') is introduced based on the normal vector of the IB, n_{IB}, that passes through point P (see Figure 2.4). The resultant value enforced is then calculated via

$$\Phi_P = C_0 + n_{IB} \cdot \nabla\Phi_{IB} x'_P + C_1 y'_P + C_2 x'_P y'_P + C_3 (x'_P)^2 + C_4 (y'_P)^2. \tag{2.15}$$

The surface of an immersed geometry may now be very complicated. Nonetheless, if the resolution of the underlying structured grid is sufficient, results close to the surface remain accurate [61]. Moreover, Ye et al. [114] show that this kind of procedures yield a discretisation error which is proportional to the square of the grid size (second order accuracy), if the underlying spatial discretisation of the partial differential equation is of at least second order. In the special case of moving immersed walls, the resultant method is sometimes called Eulerian-Lagrangian but should not be confused with the previously described ALE formulation. Here, the grid remains fully stationary Eulerian, but the walls are tracked in a Lagrangian fashion [61]. This way the governing Equations (2.3) and (2.5) remain unchanged and no additional computational costs have to be spent for mesh motion determination.

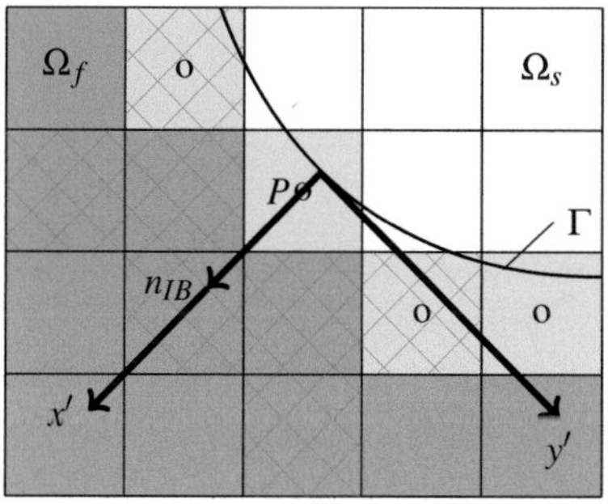

Figure 2.4: Schematic sketch of the grid separation and the interpolation procedure for imposing boundary conditions at an immersed surface. Sketch adapted from Tuković [99].

2.3.3 Fluid-Structure Interaction

FSI in the heart occurs between the blood flow and the heart's wall and valves. While the heart wall's movement represents the driving force which keeps the blood flowing, the heart valves move due to the blood's shear and pressure forces acting on them. Nonetheless, in both cases, the shear and pressure forces act from the fluid on the solids and the resultant wall movements influence the flow. Thus, these quantities have to be exchanged on the coupling interface [39].

Typically, a no-slip condition has to be fulfilled at the interface, yielding that the blood velocity, u_i, has to be equal to the velocity of the solid, v_i,

$$u_i = v_i. \tag{2.16}$$

The surface forces per unit area, $\sigma_{ij,s}$, acting on the solid surface with normal vector n_j, are composed of the pressure forces and the friction forces exerted by the blood, i.e.

$$\sigma_{ij,s}n_j = -pn_j + \tau_{ij}n_j. \tag{2.17}$$

Only time-dependent FSI problems are considered in the present work. If the solution is available at time t, then the solution at time $t+\Delta t$ is dependent on the solution of each sub-problem as well as on their interaction. There exist two approaches to tackle this task: the monolithic and the partitioned approach. They are schematically shown in Figure 2.5. The monolithic formulation assumes that fluid and solid can be seen as one continuum instead of two separated domains. Thus, only one system of equations exists, where the boundary conditions are not exchanged at an interface but are directly included. The whole system is solved at once [38, 39]. In the partitioned formulation the two domains of fluid and solid remain separated and are solved separately. Loose and strong coupling schemes are distinguished. For loose coupling, the solutions available at time t serve as boundary conditions for the next time step [39], indicated by the arrows in Figure 2.5. The interaction at time $t+\Delta t$ is not taken into account. Thereby, some effects of the interaction might remain hidden. Strong coupling is achieved by iteratively solving both sets of equations until the entire system satisfies a predefined convergence criterion. Thus, the interaction is improved which is essential for strong added-mass effects.

A good stability [39, 42] combined with a high accuracy [38] are the major advantages of choosing a monolithic approach. However, in most cases a new numerical scheme to solve the coupled system has to be developed for each specific problem [38] and it is difficult to keep the computational costs acceptable with growing complexity [42]. Applying a partitioned approach, existing solvers for fluid and structure can be chosen independently which results in higher efficiency compared to the monolithic approach [39, 42]. In terms of stability and accuracy, this method has to use smaller time steps compared to the monolithic one. It is also possible to reach a comparable accuracy, if the boundary conditions at the interface are exchanged multiple times per time step until the solutions for both systems of equations are converged [42]. This strongly coupled strategy still allows the use of different solvers for fluid and structure.

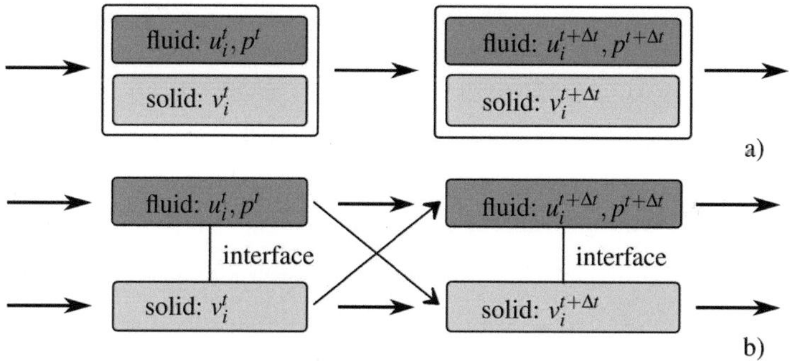

Figure 2.5: Schematic representation of solving FSI problems applying a) a monolithic and b) a partitioned approach. Sketch adapted from Hou et al. [38].

Additional disadvantages of the partitioned approach, especially in the loose coupling case, are the stability problems that occur when coupling a solid with density ρ_s and an incompressible fluid with density ρ such that $\frac{\rho_s}{\rho} \approx 1$ [42, 48]. A brief introduction to the origin of the so-called added mass effect is given in the following based on the example from Meyer (2014). Further information is provided by Tallec and Mouro [96].

A double-mass oscillator, where the mass m represents the fluid and m_s the solid, serves as example (compare Figure 2.6). At time t, a force, F, acts on the system. The analytical solution of the system results in a displacement,

$$x = \frac{F}{m + m_s} \frac{\Delta t^2}{2}. \tag{2.18}$$

The decoupled solution procedure starts with solving the translation of the solid mass. Due to the separation of the systems, the resultant solution is similar to Equation (2.18), but missing the fluid mass. The resultant displacement, x_s (compare Figure 2.6), is therefore too large.

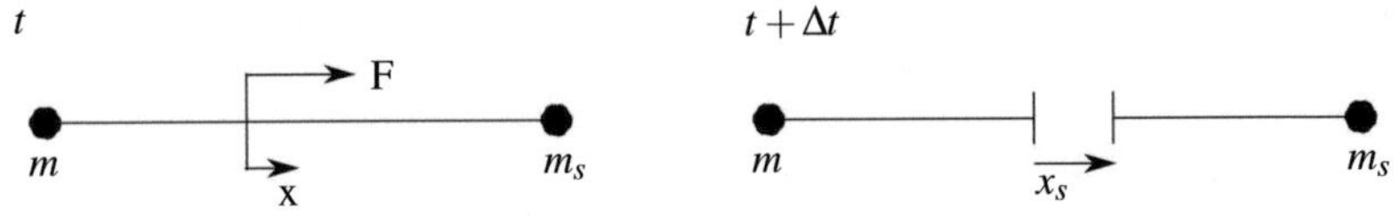

Figure 2.6: A double mass oscillator at time t and $t+\Delta t$ consisting of a fluid mass, m, and a solid mass, m_s.

In the next step, x_s serves as boundary condition for the solution of the fluid system. The solution results in a restoring force. If this restoring force is larger than the acting force, F, the system is unstable and the solution diverges. Having a look at the simplified momentum equation,

$$\rho \frac{\mathrm{d}u_i}{\mathrm{d}t} = -\frac{\mathrm{d}p}{\mathrm{d}x_i}, \tag{2.19}$$

shows that the added mass effect becomes stronger for small time steps, Δt. Further, if $\rho_s \gg \rho$, the solid mass dominates the solution of Equation (2.18) and the influence of the fluid mass becomes negligible. In the case of strong coupling, the added-mass effect is resolved and systems with low density ratios can be solved without time step restrictions.

The introduced motion techniques, namely prescription of wall movement with ALE or IBM, are solved numerically in order to describe the motion of the ventricular wall or the MV leaflets within the present work. Thus, a verification of the implementation into the solver is mandatory and presented in the following chapter. Wall movement resultant from FSI is additionally implemented and verified for future work.

3 Verification of the Numerical Procedure

In order to assure that the simulation results obtained with OpenFOAM are trustworthy the numerical procedure is tested throughout this chapter. Thereby, the tests start with a steady pipe flow and gain in complexity throughout the sections. The descriptions of solver settings, boundary conditions and meshing details ought to enable reproducibility. However, the discretisation methods are not the focus of this work. An overview of the solver settings is found in Appendix A.1.

3.1 Volume Flux Preservation

Peskin [73] states that the IBM tends to violate the conservation of mass in close proximity to the immersed body's boundary. This is mainly caused by the faults made through the mapping of the boundary onto the non-body fitted grid, such that the original geometry is not properly conserved. Performing a refinement of the Eulerian grid should significantly reduce this error.

Therefore, Stark (2013) tests the conservation of mass of the IBM used in this work on the flow through three different pipe geometries, namely a straight pipe, a 45° bent pipe and a 90° bent pipe. In all three cases the fluid properties are set to be similar to a Newtonian blood model, resulting in a kinematic viscosity $\nu = 3.6 \cdot 10^{-6}\mathrm{m}^2\,\mathrm{s}^{-1}$. The pipe diameter is set close to an approximate aortic diameter of $d = 0.03$m and the pipe length is chosen to be $l = 0.1$m. In order to prevent backflow over the outlet, the bent pipes are elongated to $l = 0.15$m. Along the immersed pipe wall the no-slip condition is enforced. In all three cases, a parabolic 3D velocity profile, based on the analytical solution for a fully developed laminar pipe flow, is prescribed at the inlet, while a fixed reference pressure, $p = 0$, is set at the outlet. Three different bulk Reynolds numbers – $\mathrm{Re}_b = \frac{u_b d}{\nu} = 10$, $\mathrm{Re}_b = 100$ and $\mathrm{Re}_b = 1000$ – are realised based on the bulk (mean) velocity, u_b. Further, two different mesh levels are examined. The base mesh consists of 50 structured hexahedral cells per 0.1m base pipe length in each direction, indexed by the fraction $\frac{1}{50}$ in Table 3.1. Close to the immersed boundary a mesh refinement is applied, which refines the mesh in all directions by a factor of two. The next finer mesh level, indexed by a factor of $\frac{1}{100}$ results in cells of half the size compared to the first configuration. Associated sketches of the three pipe geometries immersed into the corresponding meshes can be seen in Figure 3.1.

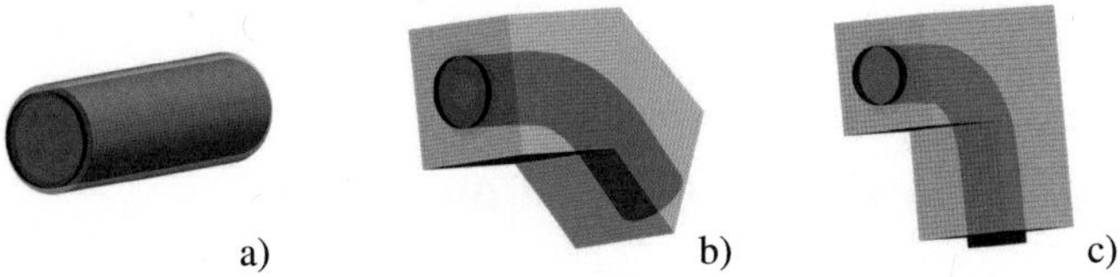

Figure 3.1: Pipe geometries immersed into structured hexahedral meshes with different curvatures: a) straight, b) 45° bent, c) 90° bent.

Based on the presented simple configurations it is possible to demonstrate the reliability of the implemented IBM in terms of mass conservation for a variety of laminar applications, as they include the range of pure shear in case of the straight pipe up to direct impact in case of the 90° bent pipe. Stark (2013) uses first-order discretisation schemes.

Table 3.1 shows the percentage of the deviation of volume flux, $\dot{V}$, at the pipe outlet compared to the prescribed volume flux at the pipe inlet for all discussed cases. It can be seen that the deviations in the cases of a straight pipe are independent of Re_b and always below 0.3%. Thus, the IBM, as realised in OpenFOAM-1.6-ext and foam-extend 3.1, is capable to compute reliable flow results in terms of pure shear at laminar Re_b. If the pipe is bent, increased deviations are found, especially in terms of the largest flow rate. As such, care has to be taken in cases, where direct flow impact is expected at the immersed boundary. Nonetheless, a mesh refinement results in sufficiently small errors in terms of volume flux deviations with respect to the desired application (compare Table 3.1).

pipe configuration	**mesh level**	**deviation of $\dot{V}$ [%]**		
		$\mathrm{Re}_b = 10$	$\mathrm{Re}_b = 100$	$\mathrm{Re}_b = 1000$
straight	$\frac{1}{50}$	0.25	0.25	0.25
	$\frac{1}{100}$	0.2	0.2	0.2
45° bent	$\frac{1}{50}$	0.08	0.05	1.7
	$\frac{1}{100}$	0.2	0.25	0.03
90° bent	$\frac{1}{50}$	1.6	2.3	6.6
	$\frac{1}{100}$	0.3	0.07	1.5

Table 3.1: Mass conservation in different pipe geometries using the IBM.

Transferring the results to the application of prescribed wall motion, the mesh resolution has to be adapted accordingly to the motion velocity. Otherwise, the mass conservation over the whole system cannot be guaranteed, as the resulting flow perpendicular to the immersed boundary is not properly captured. As such, a simulation using the IBM needs smaller cell sizes compared to the ALE formulation.

3.2 Prescription of Wall Movement

In contrast to the ALE formulation, the underlying mesh is not altered, when the immersed body is moved. Nonetheless, the movement results in changes of the fluid volume within the IB cells which has to be taken into account when the continuity equation is solved. Figure 3.2 shows two possible control volume specifications for a near-wall cell, where the right wall is moving with a constant speed, U_{out}, resulting in an additional volume, ΔV, after the regarded time, Δt. The system is comparable to a moving piston. With respect to a moving mesh, the dashed control volume is comparable to a near-wall cell that grows in dependence of the wall movement. In an IBM framework, the control volume is comparable to the fluid portion within an IB cell which also grows with the moving wall even though the total cell volume is preserved. It is assumed that no fluxes cross the upper and lower boundary in any case. The inlet velocity, U_{in}, necessary to fulfil the continuity equation is to be found. The following two analytical approaches are possible to solve the underlying problem:

1. A quasi-steady system is assumed, where the control volume marked with dashed lines in Figure 3.2 does not change its size. The movement of the piston is modelled by an outflow velocity, U_{out}, across the eastern wall of the control volume (compare Figure 3.2 a)).
2. The eastern wall moves within the regarded time with the piston and thus changes the size of the control volume by ΔV (see Figure 3.2 b)).

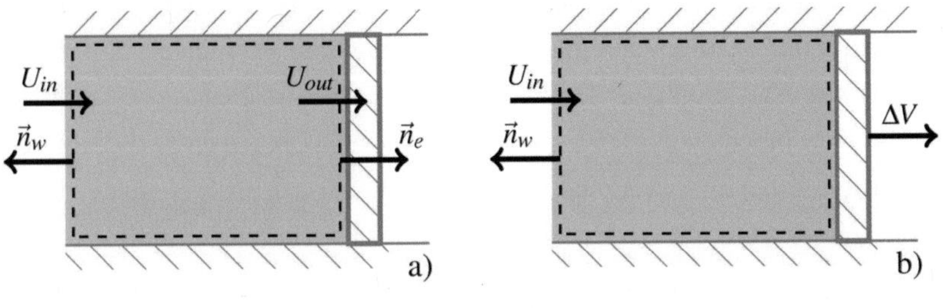

Figure 3.2: Two possibilities of defining a control volume in case of a moving boundary, where a) the volume change is taken into account via an outflow velocity, U_{out}, and b) the control volume changes its size by ΔV.

To find U_{in}, the continuity equation, Equation (2.1), is integrated over the control volume, V, such that

$$\iiint\limits_V \frac{\partial \rho}{\partial t} \mathrm{d}V = - \iiint\limits_V \frac{\partial (\rho u_i)}{\partial x_i} \mathrm{d}V. \tag{3.1}$$

In the first case, the quasi steady control volume, the time derivative in the first term of Equation (3.1) is zero. Using the Gauß integral theorem, the volume integral can be transformed into a surface integral over the control volume boundaries. The derivative is then replaced by a multiplication with the boundary normal vector, n_i, which points outwards of the control volume (compare Figure 3.2). Solving the surface integral results in the sum of all mass fluxes that pass through the respective boundaries. Inserting the assumed constant velocity distributions, normal vectors $\vec{n_w}$ and $\vec{n_e}$, and boundary area A for the control volume in Figure 3.2, leads to U_{in} being equal to the prescribed outlet velocity. Hence, the continuity of the system is fulfilled:

$$\begin{aligned} 0 &= - \iint\limits_A \rho u_i n_i \mathrm{d}A, \\ 0 &= \rho U_{in} A - \rho U_{out} A, \\ U_{out} &= U_{in}. \end{aligned} \tag{3.2}$$

In the second case with changing control volume, the time derivative cannot be eliminated. Instead, it results in the mass inserted into the system by the changing volume. The sum over all mass fluxes this time only results in one term generated by the inlet velocity:

$$\begin{aligned} \rho \tfrac{\Delta V}{\Delta t} &= - \iint\limits_A \rho u_i n_i \mathrm{d}A, \\ \rho U_{out} A &= \rho U_{in} A, \\ U_{out} &= U_{in}. \end{aligned} \tag{3.3}$$

Obviously, this approach analytically leads to the same results as the previous one. However, an extraction of the term $\rho U_{out} A$ yields the opposite sign as it is located on the opposite side of the equation. It is important to note that prior to the identification of this meaningful difference the simulation results with the IBM solver led to solver divergence or wrongly oriented velocity vectors and fluctuating pressure fields. In the original IBM toolkit available for OpenFOAM-1.6-ext, the divergence at the IB is evaluated based on Equation (3.2). However, Equation (3.3) should be applied in the case of a moving boundary to assure a proper flux direction.

The corrected implementation of the IBM with moving boundaries is tested on three different geometries (compare Figure 3.3). For comparison and verification, the test cases are additionally solved in an ALE configuration. All cases consist of four walls, where the upper wall represents the inlet and the lower wall moves downwards. Thereby, the volume increases and a volume flux equal to the volume change adjusts through the inlet. The side walls are set to be free of friction to avoid discontinuities in the corners.

Three different moving wall configurations are chosen to determine the performance of the IBM in cases where

a) the moving wall is oriented parallel to the cell faces such that all IB cells contain equal fluid volume and all IB cells have to be re-evaluated at once when the wall travels past them,

b) the moving wall is inclined such that the IB cells are still divided by a straight cut into fluid portion and structure portion but the interpolation of cell values and gradients is not straightforward because the boundary normal vector is not pointing perpendicular to the direction of motion,

c) the moving wall is curved based on a sine wave to test the interpolation of values and gradients in the IB cells with a complex boundary configuration, e.g. following a curved heart wall.

Cells sizes are designed to be equidistant hexahedral at initialisation of the flat wall case such that $\Delta x = \Delta y$. The distribution of cells is adapted in the two other cases resulting in the same number of cells. The bottom wall is moved using the shifted cosine function shown in Table 3.2. Thereby, a velocity jump is induced after initialisation followed by a smooth acceleration and deceleration such that different motion configurations are covered. These tests originate from the challenge to fulfil the continuity equation in case the boundary is moving. The transport parameters listed in Table 3.2 are chosen according to tutorial case set-ups found in the foam-extend 3.1 tutorials that are known to function in a steady state scenario. It has to be noted that the stabilisation of the calculation is more demanding if the viscosity is decreased so as to represent blood viscosity.

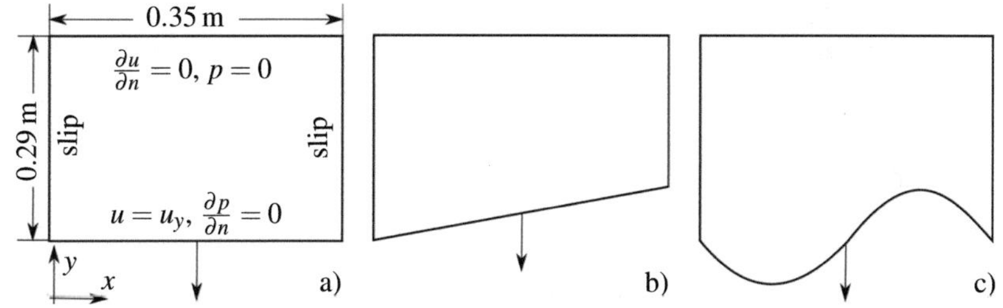

Figure 3.3: Three 2D test cases for validating moving mesh solvers. The lower wall with different shapes – a) flat, b) inclined, c) curvilinear – is moved such that the volume of the geometry increases.

$u_y[\mathrm{m\,s^{-1}}]$	$\nu[\mathrm{m^2\,s^{-1}}]$	$\Delta t[\mathrm{s}]$	$CFL_{max}[-]$	$\Delta x[\mathrm{m}]$
$-5.6 \cdot 10^{-4}(\cos(2\pi t + \pi) + 1)$	0.003	0.01	0.44	0.005

Table 3.2: Simulation settings used in the moving boundary test cases.

All simulations are examined for one half period such that the velocity starts and ends without acceleration. Figure 3.4 shows the resultant volume flux, $\dot{V}_{in}$, for all cases and the corresponding deviation from the analytical solution. The compliance of the results is high and only one volume flux curve is visually seen. Regarding the resultant deviations, the IBM results displayed in dashed lines all show equally low errors while the ALE results displayed in solid lines appear more disordered. The initial discontinuity of the velocity results in the highest deviation. Nonetheless, the solver is able to quickly capture the discrepancy and the error reduces with time. In general, both solvers are able to reproduce the analytical solution and minimise errors to below 1 %.

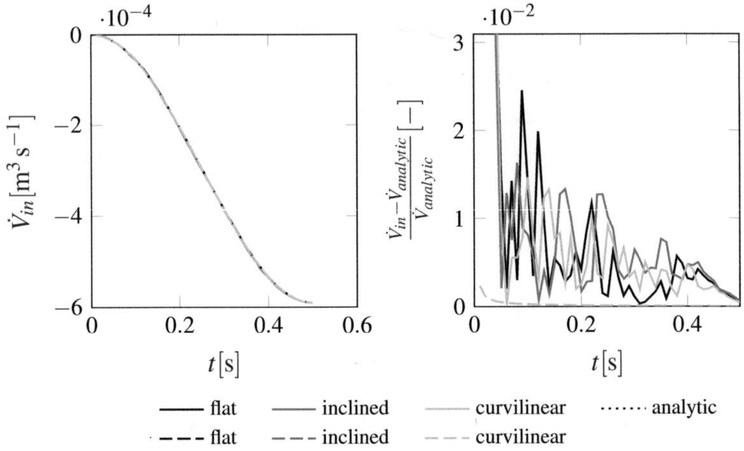

Figure 3.4: (left) Results of volume flux test cases using (solid lines) an ALE configuration and (dashed lines) an IBM configuration. (right) Resulting volume fluxes are compared to the analytic solution.

3.3 Fluid-Structure Interaction

The foam-extend 3.1 solver that enables the solution of FSI problems in combination with the IBM was developed in cooperation with Associate Professor Tuković, Professor Jasak and Damir Rigler from the Chair of Turbomachinery at the University of Zagreb, Croatia. It is based on the FSI solver distributed with foam-extend 3.1 which originally uses an ALE framework. Thus, the official FSI solver is expanded with an IBM flow solver that allows a moving boundary. The solver is currently not available in any official OpenFOAM distribution. Both, fluid and solid, are solved with the finite-volume method. For more information on the solid mechanics solution with the finite-volume method it is referred to the corresponding literature [13]. First tests showed that the challenges with respect to the continuity equation are negligible if the solid is incompressible and fully immersed into the fluid. In this case, the fluxes generated by moving walls facing each other sum up to zero. The performance of the newly established solver is briefly tested in the following.

Figure 3.5 pictures the geometric set-up of a numerical FSI test case proposed by Hron and Turek [39]. The black cylinder is rigid while the grey beam is elastic and follows the Saint Venant-Kirchhoff material law. A parabolic velocity profile is prescribed at the inlet. The Newtonian fluid flow develops vortex shedding at the tip of the beam which enhances a swinging motion of the flexible beam. For comparison with the reference data, the motion of the beam tip is recorded.

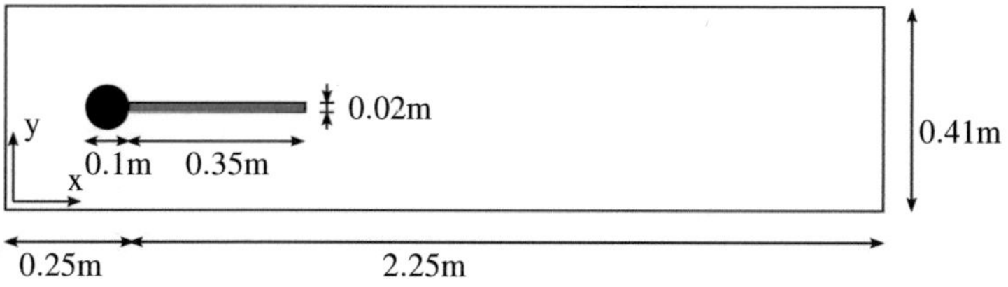

Figure 3.5: Geometric specifications of the FSI benchmark suggested by Hron and Turek [39].

Three different test scenarios are created by changing the parameter settings as listed in Table 3.3. Therein, ν_s denotes the Poisson ratio and μ_s denotes the shear modulus of the structure. In the first test case (FSI1), the bulk velocity of the flow is too low to enhance a swinging motion of the beam and the solver converges to a steady solution. The test cases FSI2 and FSI3 both result in a tip oscillation where the first responds with a lower amplitude but higher frequency compared to the latter one (compare Figure 3.6). An implicit coupling by means of the Aitken relaxation is chosen to achieve a stable and accurate coupling between fluid and solid despite the critical density ratios. Thereby, the relaxation factor varies dynamically throughout the iterations within a time step based on a linear combination of the current and the previous solution. More detailed information can be found in [19, 51].

	FSI1	FSI2	FSI3
$\rho_s[10^3 \mathrm{kg\,m^{-3}}]$	1	10	1
$\nu_s[-]$	0.4	0.4	0.4
$\mu_s[10^6 \mathrm{kg\,m^{-1}\,s^{-2}}]$	0.5	0.5	2
$\rho[10^3 \mathrm{kg\,m^{-3}}]$	1	1	1
$\nu[10^{-3} \mathrm{m^2\,s^{-1}}]$	1	1	1
$u_b[\mathrm{m\,s^{-1}}]$	0.2	1	2

Table 3.3: Simulation settings for FSI test cases chosen in accordance with Hron and Turek [39].

Figure 3.6 shows the y-displacement of the beam tip for the reference case and two different mesh configurations, where the beam is immersed into the structured mesh and the cylinder mesh is body conformal. The coarser mesh contains 5418 fluid cells and 630 solid cells. The cells are halved in both directions in the refined case, leading to 21484 fluid cells and 2520 solid cells. Resulting deviations compared to the literature are found in Table 3.4. In terms of FSI2, the mesh refinement does not improve the solution. However, the solution based on the coarse mesh is already good. With respect to FSI3, the coarse mesh results in a tip displacement amplitude that is 25 % off compared to the reference. In contrast, the corresponding frequency is close to the reported result. Here, the mesh refinement yields a significant improvement.

Solving the same test cases with equivalent mesh and solver settings, the ALE solver results in similar trends. A mesh refinement does not improve the solution in the FSI2 case, while a mesh refinement is necessary in the FSI3 case.

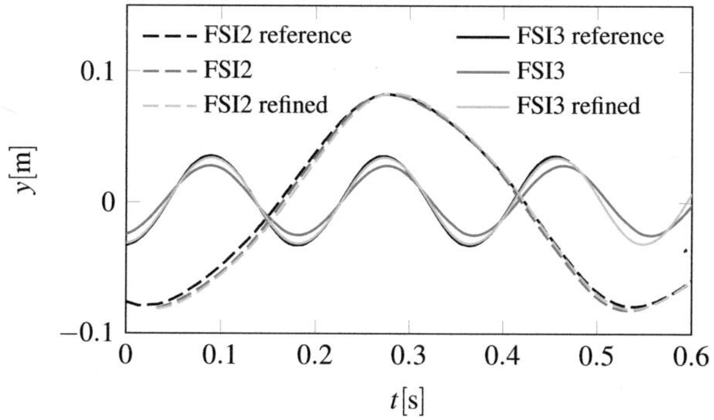

Figure 3.6: Resulting tip displacement in y-direction of the FSI test cases.

	IBM		ALE	
	amplitude	frequency	amplitude	frequency
FSI2, coarse	2.5 %	1.7 %	8.8 %	2.8 %
FSI2, fine	1.7 %	2.5 %	8.8 %	2.8 %
FSI3, coarse	25 %	2.5 %	13 %	1 %
FSI3, fine	4.2 %	0.28 %	1.2 %	0.03 %

Table 3.4: Resulting deviations of the FSI test cases compared to Hron and Turek [39].

Summarising the results, the IBM solver is capable to reliably reproduce the FSI test case and shows a similar performance as the ALE solver on equivalent meshes. Large displacements are known to challenge a numerical solver. As the higher density ratio in FSI2 reduces the added mass effects (see Chapter 2.3.3), the larger amplitude is reliably reproduced. Lowering the density ratio in FSI3 significantly increases the numerical instabilities. However, an appropriate mesh refinement enables good reproduction of the reference literature solution. The FSI1 case results in stable steady state configurations for all tested solvers and meshes.

After the validation of the numerical solver, the simulation has to be set up. Steps included in the process are the determination of material parameters, the definition of flow conditions and the geometry construction. These steps often include simplifications in numerical haemodynamics compared to the physiology of the human heart. In the following chapter pro and contra of the simplifications are summarised and evaluated.

4 Validity of Common Simplifications in Haemodynamics

During the pre-processing of a CFD case, the mathematical description of the flow case has to be determined, simulation strategies and software tools have to be chosen, material properties have to be defined, the geometry has to be constructed, and meaningful boundary conditions need to be found. The NSE (2.5) were identified in Chapter 2.2 as the partial differential equations that describe the blood flow in the human heart. In Chapter 3 the chosen solvers were tested and successfully verified. Prior to the examination of suitable boundary conditions, the validity of common simplifications in terms of material properties, the expected flow states and geometrical challenges are discussed throughout the next sections.

4.1 Non-Newtonian Fluid Properties

Blood is often modelled as incompressible Newtonian fluid [24, 71, 77, 110]. As mentioned in Chapter 2.2, the assumption of incompressibility is valid. Modelling blood as a Newtonian fluid yields that the viscosity is constant, which is true for the plasma that occupies 50 to 60% of the blood volume [3]. The plasma is in suspension with different types of cells, namely the red blood cells, the platelets and the white cells. The deformable red bloods cells that cover 95% of all cells are responsible for the non-Newtonian blood behaviour. At low shear rates ($< 1\mathrm{s}^{-1}$) they agglomerate in rolls which leads to a raise in blood viscosity. At high shear rates ($> 10\mathrm{s}^{-1}$) no agglomeration occurs but the red blood cells align and deform with the strongest shear rate direction and the blood viscosity is reduced (compare Figure 4.1) [3]. Agglomeration also vanishes when the amount of red cells in the blood, called heamatocrit, is weak ($\sim 20\%$). Further, the approximation of blood as a Newtonian fluid holds true for the quasi-steady flow in large arteries [24]. Here, the viscosity is not altered, because the shear rate is nearly constant.

Evaluating the flow through the chambers of the human heart does not include small vessels, but the flow is pulsating and thereby altering between peak values and nearly resting velocity. In the valve areas the blood is additionally subjected to sudden changes in direction and thus the velocity gradients and consequently the shear rate rise. However, Nordsletten et al. [68] state that the blood behaviour becomes approximately linear as the non-linearity develops asymptotically due to the summation of different influences, i.e. the ventricular size, the magnitude of the rate-of-strain tensor, the invariance of red blood cell concentration, and the frequency of the heart beat. With respect to these influences, Long et al. [56] state that the assumption of blood being Newtonian in the heart is valid as long as the blood is in movement. Towards the end of the systole and the end of the diastole, the shear rate decreases and non-Newtonian effects might occur.

Amblard et al. [3] highlight that in zones where the local haemodynamics are disturbed, non-Newtonian effects also play an important role, e.g. in endoprosthesis or around the heart valve tips. They adapt the Phan-Thien and Tanner model [97], which is based on the theory of networks. Originally developed for studying lubricants, the tangle of polymers represents the aggregation and dislocation of the red cells. The reported results for abdominal aortic aneurysms look promising. Nonetheless, the model is not tested in a ventricular geometry and the solution of an additional differential equation increases the computational costs in comparison to a Newtonian model.

An easy approach that does not introduce additional computational costs is to use a phenomenological model, e.g. Bingham, Casson, Ostwald de Waele, Prandtl-Eyring or Sisko. These models incorporate non-Newtonian behaviour but treat blood as a homogeneous fluid. The incompressible, Newtonian solver can easily be adapted by replacing the effective viscosity, μ_{eff}, in the NSE (2.5) by a shear rate dependent viscosity.

In order to compare Newtonian and non-Newtonian descriptions at equal computational costs, the Carreau viscosity model [14] as used in [63] is chosen as non-Newtonian blood model. It defines the effective viscosity in dependency of the shear rate, $\dot{\gamma}$, and the material specific parameters $\mu_\infty, \mu_0, \lambda_f, n$, where μ_∞ and μ_0 define the lower and the upper limit of the resultant viscosity [69], i.e.

$$\mu_{eff}(\dot{\gamma}) = \mu_\infty + (\mu_0 - \mu_\infty)(1 + (\lambda_f \dot{\gamma})^2)^{\frac{n-1}{2}}. \quad (4.1)$$

The resultant slope of this material law is shown in Figure 4.1 as well as the blood viscosity as reported by Amblard et al. [3]. All parameters are chosen similar to the ones chosen by Mühlhausen [63] and are found in Table 4.1.

	μ_∞[Pa s]	μ_0[Pa s]	λ_f[s]	n[−]	ρ[kg m^{-3}]
Mühlhausen [63]	0.003	0.01315	0.4	0.4	1055
Gijsen et al. [29]	0.0022	0.022	0.11	0.392	1410
Amblard [3]	0.005	0.05	-	-	-

Table 4.1: Material parameters used with the Carreau viscosity model and the reported viscosity slopes in Figure 4.1.

In order to judge whether it is necessary to adopt a non-Newtonian viscosity model for heart flow simulations, Gollub (2013) presents two test cases. The first test case is a steady pipe flow and the second test case is a periodically pulsating flow in a bent pipe adapted from Gijsen et al. [30].

The basic test cases shall answer two questions. Firstly, how significant are the differences between Newtonian and non-Newtonian fluid models and secondly, whether the numerical solver determines the velocity profiles correctly.

For a fully developed pipe flow, an analytical solution for the resulting Newtonian velocity profile can be derived. Therefore, the NSE in cylindrical coordinates for the flow component $u(r)$, r being the radial coordinate, has to be solved [93]:

$$0 = -\frac{\partial p}{\partial x} + \mu_{eff}\left(\frac{\partial^2 u}{\partial r^2} + \frac{1}{r}\frac{\partial u}{\partial r}\right). \tag{4.2}$$

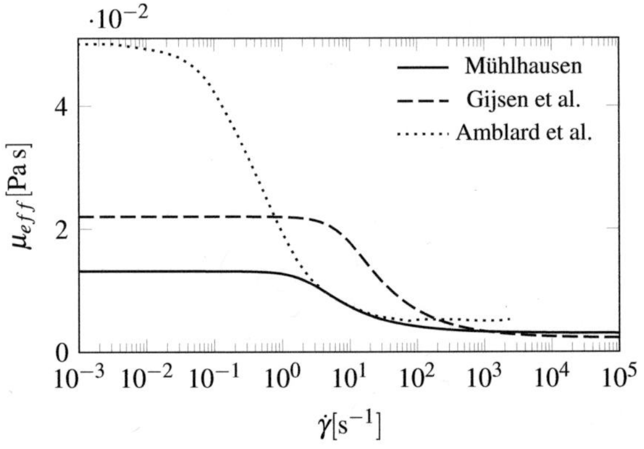

Figure 4.1: Slope of the Carreau viscosity model using the parameters in Table 4.1.

With the condition that the continuity equation is fulfilled the velocity vanishes at the pipe wall ($u(r = R) = 0$) and the shear stress vanishes at the pipe centre:

$$\tau = \mu_{eff}\left.\frac{\partial u}{\partial r}\right|_{r\to 0} = 0. \tag{4.3}$$

The solution of the Newtonian parabolic velocity profile with constant viscosity ($\mu_{eff} = \mu$) is then determined as

$$u(r) = \frac{R^2}{4\mu}\frac{\mathrm{d}p}{\mathrm{d}x}\left(1 - \frac{r^2}{R^2}\right). \tag{4.4}$$

The non-Newtonian velocity profile is calculated using a MATLAB® tool provided by Binous [9], where a system of equations build by Equation (4.1), (4.2) and (4.3) is solved numerically. Therein, μ_{eff} depends on the shear rate and thus on the pipe radius. Gollub (2013) gives a detailed description of the tools and set-ups used. The results are summarised in the following.

As the velocity profile for the non-Newtonian fluid is assumed to be unknown, the simulations are driven by a prescribed pressure gradient, such that $\mathrm{Re}_b \approx 1000$ holds for the resultant bulk Reynolds number based on the lower limit viscosity μ_∞. The maximum resulting shear rates lie at $\dot{\gamma} = 22.5\,\mathrm{s}^{-1}$ which is located in the regime of changing viscosity. In the regarded Reynolds regime and in the idealised steady configuration, the non-Newtonian model yields a flatter, yet parabolic, velocity profile compared to the Newtonian model. The difference between the respective bulk velocities is below 3 %. By altering the flow speed it is possible to generate flow scenarios with shear rates below $1\,\mathrm{s}^{-1}$, where the resulting velocity profiles are equivalent. For the pipe flow, this state is reached when the Reynolds number is decreased to 100. As seen in Figure 4.1, the limiting viscosities are not consistently chosen in the literature, as they also vary from patient to patient and can further change depending on the health status. Therefore, each group defines their own parameters.

To better understand the model characteristics with its advantages and disadvantages, an unsteady pulsating flow through a bent pipe is simulated by Gollub (2013) and compared qualitatively to the experimental and numerical results of Gijsen et al. [29]. The model parameters are adapted to fit the literature data and are found in Table 4.1. The resulting slope of the effective viscosity is found in Figure 4.1. The resulting unsteady flow profiles are significantly different in the centre of the pipe but show a similar progression towards the pipe walls. Therefore, also the results for the wall shear stress are congruent. These differences result from the differing development of the secondary flow in radial direction which is observed to be slower in the case of the non-Newtonian fluid. A major drawback of the test case is existent in the rigid wall of the geometry. In a physiological artery, the wall moves with the pressure wave and thus stores kinetic energy. It is questionable if the non-Newtonian model can react properly or rather physiologically to this event. As such, referring to the respective arguments, it is possible to approve or disapprove non-Newtonian modelling.

Every model is developed to describe the behaviour of a specific fluid. The phenomenological ones are not designed to imitate the blood viscosity. In contrast, the Phan-Thien and Tanner model is specifically designed to describe blood flow behaviour. However, it is computationally expensive. In clinical practice medical imaging information is used as basis for the shear stress determination. Blood is then treated as a Newtonian fluid [3]. Summarising all considerations it is chosen to stick to a Newtonian formulation as it is comparable to clinical results, inexpensive and the error influence of the non-Newtonian models cannot be reliably estimated.

4.2 Transition to Turbulence

It is known that the flow in the human heart can undergo transition from the laminar to the turbulent state when the incoming jet of blood impacts into the nearly resting fluid in the chamber [2, 21, 23, 53, 57]. The presence of turbulence enhances the mixing in a fluid but also increases the shear forces. Although mixing is favourable in the heart, an elevated friction rises the risk of platelet activation and haemolysis [2, 23]. Luckily, turbulence in the healthy heart hardly develops and if so remains very low. Higher or persistent existence of turbulence can be an indicator of heart diseases especially connected to small Strouhal numbers, $\mathrm{St} \leq 0.05$ [21]. This dimensionless number is based on a characteristic length, L_c, equal to the ventricular diameter, a characteristic velocity, U_c, equal to the peak flow velocity and a characteristic time scale, T_c, equal to the duration of one heart beat. Thus, a larger ventricle with slow velocities is favourable in terms of stability of the laminar flow state.

As turbulence is not expected to be present throughout the whole heart cycle, it is of special interest to detect regions where the flow might undergo transition. Further, it is important to understand the influence of different flow models on the strain and stress levels in order to assess the uncertainty of the numerical results [2]. A detailed description of the physics behind the transition process can be found in [83]. Further reading on internal transitional processes in a pipe is provided in [64, 113].

One possibility to simulate transition is to carry out direct numerical simulations (DNS) as found for example in [21, 23, 53, 57]. However, DNS are time consuming and require much larger meshes compared to laminar simulations. Thus, a realisation within the clinical practice is questionable. Chnafa et al. [15] perform the cheaper large-eddy simulation and observe that a fully turbulent state is never reached throughout the whole heart cycle. Another, even cheaper, alternative to DNS is the Reynolds-Averaged Navier-Stokes (RANS) approach. Al-Azawy et al. [2] show that in an unsteady pulsating flow through a ventricular assist device, the results obtained by a laminar approach are nearly identical to the ones obtained by the k-ω-SST model. Vellguth (2017) compares the pressure drop over the MV obtained by a laminar solver and a k-ϵ model for different levels of activity. She concludes that the influence of present turbulence is negligible. However, those RANS models cannot capture transition and treat the flow as fully turbulent.

Walters and Cokljat [106] developed a RANS model, the k-k_l-ω model, that is able to reproduce the transition from laminar to turbulent flow for external flows. The principle is outlined in the following.

The decomposition of a flow quantity, ϕ, into its time-average value, $\bar{\phi}$, and its time-dependent fluctuation value, ϕ', as

$$\phi(x_i,t) = \bar{\phi}(x_i) + \phi'(x_i,t), \tag{4.5}$$

is called Reynolds decomposition. The basic equations for RANS are determined by inserting the Reynolds decomposition into the NSE (2.5). Temporal averaging of the result yields

$$\bar{u}_j \frac{\partial \bar{u}_i}{\partial x_j} = -\frac{1}{\bar{\rho}} \frac{\partial \bar{p}}{\partial x_i} + \frac{\partial}{\partial x_j} \Bigg(\nu \frac{\partial \bar{u}_i}{\partial x_j} - \underbrace{\overline{u_i' u_j'}}_{\substack{\textit{Reynolds} \\ \textit{stresses}}} \Bigg) + f_i. \tag{4.6}$$

This procedure introduces an additional non-linear term to the right hand side of Equation (4.6) called the Reynolds stress term which introduces six additional unknowns into the system of equations. A typical way to close the system is the introduction of the Boussinesq hypothesis which assumes isotropy of the turbulence. Thereby, the six unknowns are reduced down to one via

$$\overline{u_i' u_j'} = -\nu_T \left(\frac{\partial \bar{u}_i}{\partial x_j} + \frac{\partial \bar{u}_j}{\partial x_i} \right), \tag{4.7}$$

where ν_T is called turbulent eddy viscosity.

The k-k_l-ω model is a three-equation model that introduces three transport equations as basis for the determination of ν_T: one for the laminar kinetic energy k_l, one for the turbulent kinetic energy k_T and one for the specific dissipation rate ω. An overview of the equations, the most influencing parameters and model verification is given in Appendix A.3. Detailed descriptions can be found in [106] and Klatt (2015).

Walters and Cokljat test the k-k_l-ω model on a flat plate test case and thereby prove its ability of correctly representing the transition from laminar to turbulent behaviour for external flows [105]. As the purpose of this work is the simulation of blood flow within the human heart, a different test case is considered that shall represent the transition of internal flows. Therefore, Klatt (2015) computes the friction coefficient of pipe flows with different Re_b using the k-k_l-ω model and compares the results to experimental data as well as laminar and turbulent correlations. For all cases where $\mathrm{Re}_b \leq 5000$ the same structured hexahedral mesh is used, while for $\mathrm{Re}_b > 5000$ custom meshes are created for each case. For further details on the test case set-up, refer to Klatt (2015). The results are shown in Figure 4.2.

The laminar correlation is based on the analytical solution of a fully developed pipe flow, where the pressure drop, $\frac{\mathrm{d}p}{\mathrm{d}x}$, is connected to the bulk velocity, u_b, via the Darcy friction factor, f_D:

$$-\frac{\mathrm{d}p}{\mathrm{d}x} = \frac{f_D}{d}\frac{\rho}{2}u_b^2, \tag{4.8}$$

where d is the pipe diameter. Inserting this relation into the parabolic Hagen-Poiseuille profile yields a linear function for f_D in laminar fully developed pipe flow in dependence of the Reynolds number,

$$f_D = \frac{64}{\mathrm{Re}}. \tag{4.9}$$

As turbulent correlation, the Colebrook-White equation valid for $\mathrm{Re}_b \geq 4000$ is used, where f_D is found by solving the following equation iteratively

$$\frac{1}{\sqrt{f_D}} = -2\log_{10}\left(\frac{\epsilon}{3.7d} + \frac{2.51}{\mathrm{Re}_b\sqrt{f_D}}\right). \tag{4.10}$$

A hydraulically smooth pipe is considered such that the pipe roughness is non-existent ($\epsilon = 0$) in all numerical cases. In the two presented experimental data sets, the Oregon data is measured using smooth pipes, while the Nikuradse data is measured in rough pipes and later extracted by Joseph and Yang [45] as effectively smooth data set. Both data sets are extracted from [45]. Studying Figure 4.2, it can be seen that the experimental data sets do not overlap in the linear region and also show different behaviour in the transition zone. The deviation of the Oregon data is an effect of a not fully developed pipe flow in the experimental set-up. Nonetheless, a fast and sharp transition from laminar to turbulent flow is indicated. Nikuradse does not provide data for smooth pipes in the transition zone, which might explain the deviation and smoother transition. These effects show that designing and measuring transitional effects is challenging and all results have to be interpreted with caution.

The k-k_l-ω model fits the laminar correlation with a maximum deviation of 2%. However, it follows the laminar correlation up to $\mathrm{Re}_b = 4575$ and thereby under-predicts the friction factor by up to 65% in comparison to the other available data sets. In the turbulent region higher friction factors are predicted. With an increasing Reynolds number the deviations between the different data sets decrease.

Klatt (2015) performs a new calibration of the transition model in order to improve the calculated transition point and the determined friction factor. For internal flows, the bypass transition is usually the path that the flow takes when it undergoes transition. As such, the new calibration concentrates on the term that feeds energy to the turbulent kinetic energy as soon as bypass transition is detected. Klatt (2015) identifies the model constant that is the most relevant coefficient if the effect strength of the initiated bypass transition is to be calibrated. Changing this parameter accordingly results in a shift of the transitional Reynolds number from 4600 to 3000 (compare Figure 4.2), which is in better agreement with the experimental data. Overall, the recalibrated k-k_l-ω model now predicts the friction factor too high in the turbulent regime, which is more favourable than values that are too low with respect to stress prediction in bio-mechanical flows.

Considering the request of good accuracy at low computational effort, it is yet to be shown, how the transition model performs in comparison to standard two-equation turbulence models or simple laminar calculation. Therefore, Klatt (2015) additionally compares the results to simulation results achieved with a laminar solver and with the two-equation k-ω-SST model. The choice of the latter one is based on the availability in OpenFOAM 2.3.0 and the fact that is uses the same basis framework. Figure 4.3 shows the resultant friction factor in dependency of the Reynolds number. The transition model fits very well the laminar results up to the transition point. In the turbulent region, both the k-k_l-ω model and the k-ω-SST model overestimate the friction factor at first. This overestimation decreases with an increasing Reynolds number. However, the two-equation model is closer to the measured values and the correlation.

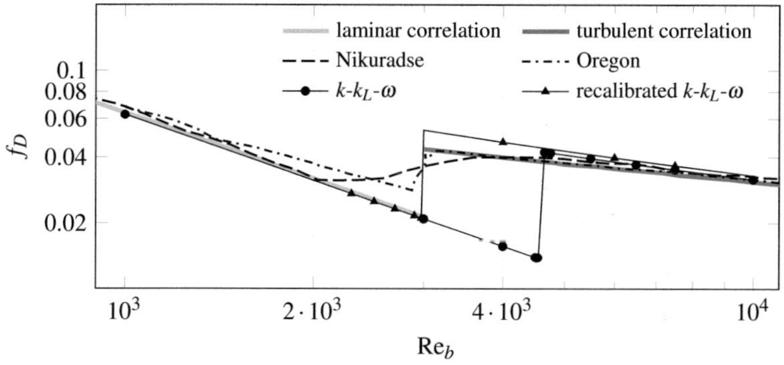

Figure 4.2: Resultant friction factor, f_D, in a pipe flow in dependency of Re_b for according correlations, literature data and different calibrations of the k-k_l-ω model.

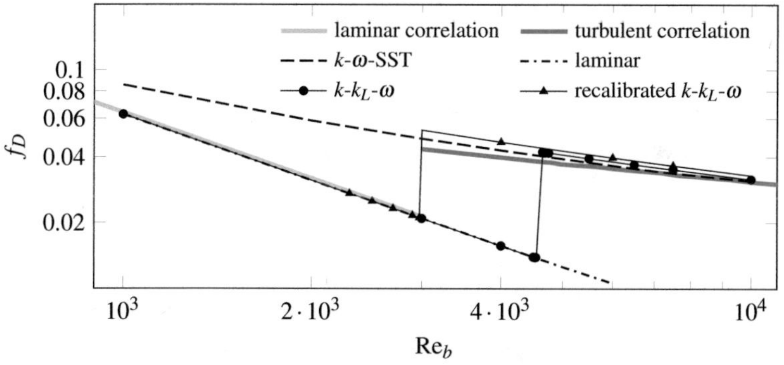

Figure 4.3: Resultant friction factor f_D in a pipe flow in dependency of Re_b for according correlations, RANS approaches and different calibrations of the k-k_l-ω model.

Klatt (2015) uses a mesh refinement study to evaluate the necessary mesh resolution for laminar simulations. He states that even for a simple pipe flow at $\mathrm{Re}_b = 1000$, the calculation using the k-k_l-ω model needs ten times more cells compared to a laminar calculation. The deviation in cell numbers even increases with an increasing Re_b. Responsible for this difference are the velocity gradients near the wall that are larger in a turbulent flow compared to a laminar flow. These gradients have to be resolved which results in a much finer mesh within the RANS framework. Even if a wall function is applied in the near-wall region, which is not appropriate in the regarded Reynolds number ranges, a sufficient resolution still results in three times more cells compared to the laminar mesh.

When using the k-ω-SST or k-k_l-ω model, two or three additional transport equations have to be solved respectively. Thus, computational effort is considerably higher in comparison to a laminar solver. At Reynolds numbers close to possible transition processes, the RANS models are not able to represent the turbulent regime. An appropriate model for bio-mechanical application in the human circulatory system should ideally be able to capture both laminar and turbulent regions. As this is not possible at a reasonable computational effort, a laminar solver is chosen in the present work over a turbulence model, especially as it is expected that the flow is mostly laminar and only undergoes transition locally and for a short time.

4.3 Geometrical Simplifications

The surface of the human LV is not smooth but covered with trabeculae (irregular muscle ridges). During the systole, they squeeze the near-wall blood and thereby support the apical washout by adding kinetic energy into the flow [103]. Rough walls enhance the generation of turbulence and increase the energy loss in terms of viscous dissipation. However, these losses are small compared to the total pressure work conducted by the pumping of the muscle. It is worth noting that the LV is the only vessel with trabeculae. Due to their squeezing mechanism, the particle residence time is equivalent to models with smooth walls such that both models are equivalently effective [103].

While the trabeculae are only present on the surface, the papillary muscles and chordae tendineae that connect the MV with the ventricular wall pass through the flow field (compare Figure 4.4) and form a blockage area that comprises about 10% of the LV volume [103]. Long et al. [56] report that small vortices form around the papillary muscles close to the inflow tract. Those small structures cannot be reproduced if the papillary muscles are neglected in CFD simulations. Regardless, large scale structures such as the main ring vortex generated during the inflow phase are similar in the measured *in-vivo* data and in the simplified CFD results [56].

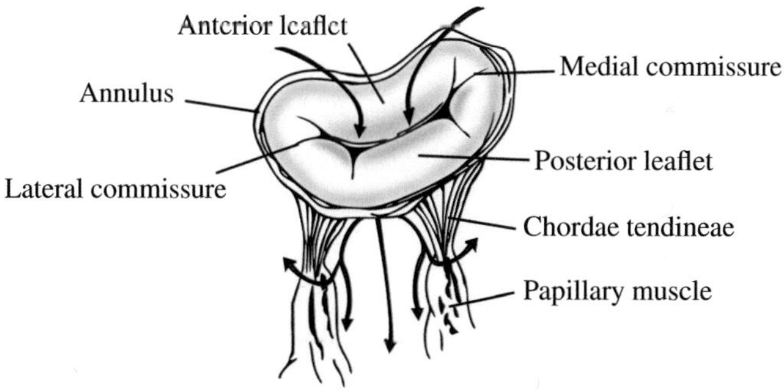

Figure 4.4: Physiological anatomy of the MV and drafted flow field vectors in case the MV opens. Sketch adapted from Iaizzo [41].

Vedula et al. [103] report significant disruption of the vortices from the early inflow phase on. Both the trabeculae and the papillary muscles are found to be responsible. The papillary muscles form recirculation zones in their wake. They provide a blockage and a guiding path for the entering jet that thereby penetrates deeper into the ventricle. An overall enhancement of the hydrodynamic efficiency in comparison to a smooth wall model is not measurable. In the LV with smooth walls, the diastolic jet travels along the posterior ventricle wall and not straight towards the apex. It has to be noted that all the observations hold for one specific patient and can vary significantly if a different heart geometry is considered. The observation outlined by Vedula et al. [103]

is that the flow characteristics in terms of jet penetration and direction as well as the vortex shape are disparate. However, measures such as residence times or the overall energy balance are comparable.

Larsson et al. [52] expand echocardiography data by CFD simulation where trabeculae, papillary muscles and valve leaflets are neglected. They state that a comparison of global flow quantities still results in correct assessment of evaluated trends. This assumption should hold true in cases where solely CFD results are compared. Besides, proper conduction of LV simulations including complex anatomical features is challenging. Available imaging techniques, e.g. echocardiography or magnetic resonance tomography, do not provide adequate temporal and spatial resolutions [77, 103]. These conclusions lead to the decision of neglecting trabeculae and papillary muscles in this work.

The complex movement of the MV leaflets is especially challenging to resolve. Thus, anatomically correct MV movement is typically neglected in CFD. It is nowadays widely accepted that the 3D leaflets play a non-negligible role when the intraventricular flow characteristics ought to be examined [7, 8]. Nonetheless, it is arguable that the leaflets mainly follow the inflowing jet and that their influence on the resulting flow field is marginal [52, 56]. Baccani et al. [7] distinguish between slow and fast valvular opening, whereby the significance of the resulting influence scales with the promptitude of the opening.

Multiple different models for dealing with the complexity of the MV have been developed in the past decades and their influences are ongoingly debated. The feasibility is not least a major challenge. An evaluation of the available MV models is conducted in Chapter 6. Before influences of the chosen MV model can be assessed, meaningful strategies and measures that reveal the fundamental differences between the models have to be identified and evaluated. Therefore, the next chapter covers the basics of the chosen vortex detection methods. Thereby, standardised criteria are established that serve as basis for the investigation of the ventricular flow field.

5 Application of Vortex Detection Methods

The vortex formation process during the diastole is the dominating flow characteristic in the heart. Size and direction of the developing structures dominate local quantities like shear-strain and also influence integral quantities such as the volume fraction. Identification and characterisation of those structures are therefore of major interest. Up to now, no universal definition of a vortex exists, although many attempts are found in the literature [27, 116].

A meaningful approach is identifying flow topologies [76] within a plane of arbitrary size and orientation. Within the plane, distinct singular points of the flow field are detected. Thereby, nodes identify vortex cores and half saddle points identify flow stagnation occurring at walls or edges. If a wall half saddle unites with a trailing edge saddle to form a full saddle, a vortex detaches from the corresponding edge. Especially for 3D flows, this method is computationally expensive and challenging to automate.

Approaches using the kinematics of the flow are based on the streamline geometry [78]. If its curvature has a well defined centre, this centre is the core of a vortex. Further improvement includes the determination of the winding-angle that also identifies weak and non-circular vortices. An automated extraction of vortex centres based on the streamline topology is proposed by Graftieaux et al. [32]. This method is applicable to 3D flows as long as the vortices project well to 2D slices through the flow field. Thus, some vortices might remain unseen. Further, the computational costs are higher compared to local Eulerian criteria.

Schlanderer (2014) compares the most widely employed local Eulerian approaches, not restricted to heart flow application. She concludes that no significant differences are found in the results due to the fact that they are all based on the vorticity vector. As the evaluation of the Q-criterion needs the least computational effort and reliably detects vortex cores, it represents the method of choice for evaluating the blood flow in the heart. Unfortunately, the Eulerian nature of this approach does not directly allow to draw conclusions regarding the time development of the flow or cause-effect relations between the identified structures.

These drawbacks are met by the application of a Lagrangian approach, where only a few are available, e.g the $\mathbf{M}_Z$-criterion [34] or detecting delocalised unsteady vortex regions [27]. The method of choice for this work is the finite-time Lyapunov exponent, which detects Lagrangian coherent structures in the flow field and thereby identifies vortex boundaries and recirculation zones. A generalised application guideline is missing in the literature for both methods, the Q-criterion and the finite-time Lyapunov exponent. Therefore, the following sections introduce the chosen vortex detection methods and provide a step towards generalisation. Excerpts of the results have been presented before [DFK16, SGK$^+$15, SSKK14].

5.1 Eulerian Approach – Q-criterion

The motion of a fluid element consists of up to four components: translation, rotation, shear-strain and dilatation. As seen in Figure 5.1, a fluid element does not change its shape under translation or rotation. These motions are called solid-body motions. In the case of shear-strain or dilatation, the faces of the fluid element move relative to each other.

Eulerian approaches of vortex identification are commonly based on the calculation of the vorticity vector ω_i and its relation to the strain vector. The vorticity is defined as the curl of the velocity and represents the rotation of a fluid element:

$$\omega_i = \epsilon_{jki} \frac{\partial u_k}{\partial x_j}. \tag{5.1}$$

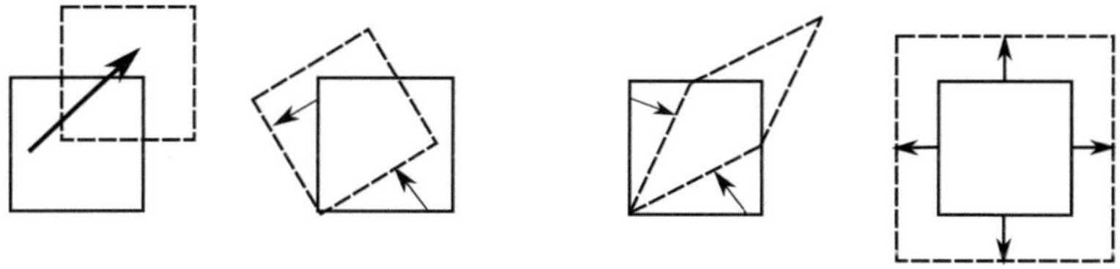

Figure 5.1: Possible components of fluid element motion. Sketch adapted from Spurk and Aksel [93].

Vorticity and strain both contribute to the velocity gradient. This is shown by splitting the velocity gradient into its antisymmetric and symmetric part, as

$$\frac{\partial u_i}{\partial x_j} = \underbrace{\frac{1}{2}\left(\frac{\partial u_i}{\partial x_j} - \frac{\partial u_j}{\partial x_i}\right)}_{\Omega_{ij}} + \underbrace{\frac{1}{2}\left(\frac{\partial u_i}{\partial x_j} + \frac{\partial u_j}{\partial x_i}\right)}_{S_{ij}} = \Omega_{ij} + S_{ij}. \tag{5.2}$$

The rate-of-strain tensor S_{ij} measures the amount of local folding and stretching of a fluid element and the rotation tensor Ω_{ij}, whose components are build of the vorticity ω_i, measures the rotation.

To clarify the origin of vorticity and strain, Figure 5.2 pictures their components. The solid rectangle, with edge lengths Δx_1 and Δx_2, represents a fluid element in the initial configuration at time t. The dashed geometry represents the deformed state at $t + \Delta t$. Thereby, the index R denotes rotation and S denotes shear-strain. Lateral displacement of the element corners, denoted by a

and b, is dependent on the respective velocity gradient acting during the time interval Δt, such that

$$a^R = a^S = \frac{\partial u_2}{\partial x_1}\Delta x_1 \Delta t; \qquad b^R = -b^S = -\frac{\partial u_1}{\partial x_2}\Delta x_2 \Delta t. \tag{5.3}$$

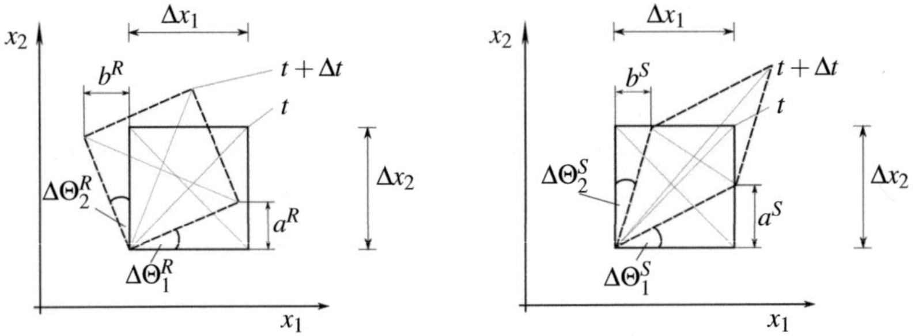

Figure 5.2: (left) Rotation and (right) shear-strain effects acting on a fluid element. Sketch adapted from Spurk and Aksel [93].

As for example shown by Schlanderer (2014), the angular velocities of the depicted fluid element can for small angular changes $\Delta\Theta$ be related to the velocity gradients by

$$\frac{d\Theta_1^R}{dt} = \frac{d\Theta_1^S}{dt} = \frac{\partial u_2}{\partial x_1}; \qquad \frac{d\Theta_2^R}{dt} = \frac{d\Theta_2^S}{dt} = -\frac{\partial u_1}{\partial x_2}. \tag{5.4}$$

Using the definitions of the rotation tensor and the rate-of-strain tensor in Equation (5.2), the respective components acting in x_3-direction are determined as

$$\Omega_{21} = \frac{1}{2}\left(\frac{d\Theta_1^R}{dt} + \frac{d\Theta_2^R}{dt}\right); \qquad S_{21} = \frac{1}{2}\left(\frac{d\Theta_1^S}{dt} - \frac{d\Theta_2^S}{dt}\right). \tag{5.5}$$

Inserting Equation (5.4) into Equation (5.5) yields the respective parts of the velocity gradient in Equation (5.2).

Hunt et al. [40] introduce the second invariant of the velocity gradient, Q, as indicator for vortices in the flow:

$$Q = \frac{1}{2}((\| \Omega_{ij} \|)^2 - (\| S_{ij} \|)^2). \tag{5.6}$$

If $Q > 0$ holds true, the rotation of a fluid element becomes dominant over the stretching and thus a vortex is found in the flow field. This principle is shown in application using an analytical 2D flow field called the double gyre. This test scenario is especially interesting for demonstrating the differences between Eulerian and Lagrangian characterisation techniques [89]. It comprises of two counter-rotating vortices that are separated by a periodically translating middle axis. The corresponding stream-function $\Theta(x,y,t)$ applied within the domain $[0,2] \times [0,1]$ is defined as

$$\Theta(x,y,t) = A\sin(\pi f(x,t))\sin(\pi y), \tag{5.7}$$

$$\text{with} \quad f(x,t) = c\sin(\omega_f \pi t)x^2 + (1 - 2c\sin(\omega_f \pi t))x. \tag{5.8}$$

The coefficients are chosen according to Shadden et al. [89] and Kaiser (2014), i.e. $A = 0.1\,\mathrm{m^2\,s^{-1}}$, $c = 0.25$ and $\omega_f = 0.2\,\mathrm{s^{-1}}$. Thus, one period lasts $10\,\mathrm{s}$. Figure 5.3 shows exemplary the double gyre flow field and the Q-criterion for two different time steps.

Decreasing the resolution of the velocity data affects the results of the Q-criterion. The contours become coarser (compare Figure 5.4). With ten velocity points along the height of the domain, the shape of the rotational zone starts looking fuzzy but still similar to the highly resolved result depicted in Figure 5.3. Further, the centres of the two identified vortices remain in the correct position. Another quartering of the velocity data results in a displacement of the vortex centres and thus a faulty detection. These observations can be related to Eulerian grid resolutions for CFD, where a resolution of ten cells is considered adequate to cover rotational movement in the flow.

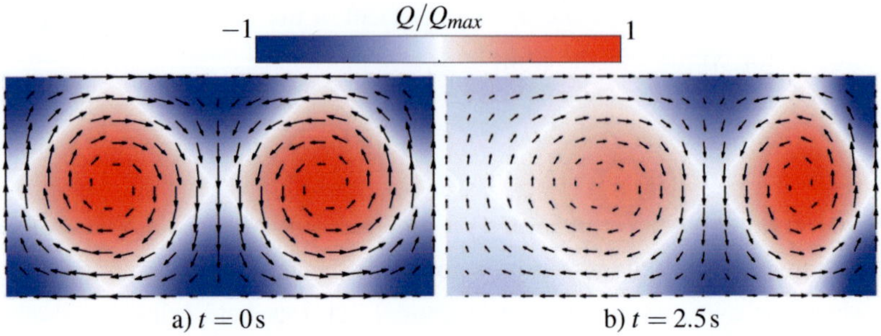

Figure 5.3: Double gyre flow (black arrows) at two different time points and the corresponding Q contour scaled by the largest value Q_{max}.

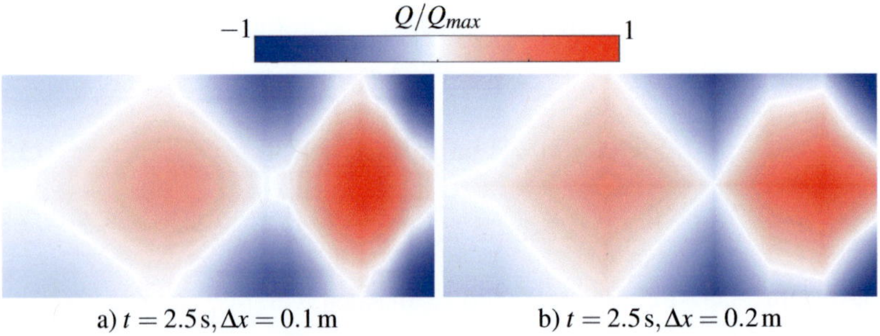

Figure 5.4: Q contour of the double gyre flow scaled by the largest value Q_{max} with decreasing mesh resolution from a) to b).

The Eulerian nature of the Q-criterion yields that only momentary information is transported. Time-dependent flow evolution cannot be covered. Thus, the time resolution of the flow field does not affect the results.

The Q-criterion if often used to visualise vortices in 3D flow fields by means of extracted iso-surfaces. Thereby, the choice of the depicted iso-value is arbitrary and no clear definition of a vortex boundary exists. Schlanderer (2014) identifies multiple dimensionless quantities that ought to relate Q to other characteristic flow quantities, e.g. bulk velocity, vorticity or a characteristic length. These number are then evaluated in different flow fields, i.e. a Rankine vortex, a 3D ring vortex and an exemplary heart flow. The purpose of this attempt is to find a critical characteristic value that provides an iso-value applicable in different kinds of rotational flows. Unfortunately, a globally applicable quantity has still to be found and case dependent Q-values are used for visualisations in this work.

5.2 Lagrangian Approach – Finite-Time Lyapunov Exponent

The identification of Lagrangian coherent structures (LCS) is a method to examine the Lagrangian behaviour of a flow field. LCS are separatrices in form of material lines (2D) or surfaces (3D) that divide the flow into areas (2D) or volumes (3D) of coherent movement. Hereby, hyperbolic LCS are defined as attracting and repelling manifolds [35], depending on whether flow particles tend to move towards or away from the LCS. These possible scenarios are schematically shown in Figure 5.5, where the repelling manifold is drawn in blue and the attracting manifold is drawn in red. LCS are mathematically derived by tracking the movement of particle clouds and evaluating the particle separation rate in terms of the finite-time Lyapunov exponent (FTLE).

Two particles x_0 and $x_0 + \delta x_0$, with infinitesimal distance δx_0, are tracked over the time span $T_{int} = t_1 - t_0$ (compare Figure 5.5). The separation rate provides information about the stability of the starting point [47]. If the separation rate is high, the stability of the starting point is low. This behaviour can be investigated forward in time ($t_0 < t_1$), revealing repelling LCS, or backward in time ($t_0 > t_1$), revealing attracting LCS.

The FTLE, $\sigma_{t_0}^{t_1}$, is defined as

$$\sigma_{t_0}^{t_1} = \lim_{\delta x_0 \to 0} \frac{1}{|T_{int}|} \ln \frac{\delta x(t_1)}{\delta x_0}. \tag{5.9}$$

It evaluates the exponential growth ratio of the distance between the two particles during the integration interval. To determine the distance at time t_1, an ordinary differential equation that describes the particle motion in the flow has to be solved. Thereby, the particle paths are determined. The resultant flow map, $\Phi_{t_0}^{t_1}$, stores the mapping that relates the initial particle position at time t_0 of each particle to its final position at time t_1. Thus, the current particle position is stored in the third-order tensor, $\Phi_{t_0}^{t_1}$, with respect to its starting position:

$$\Phi_{t_0}^{t_1} : \mathbb{R}^n \quad \longmapsto \quad \mathbb{R}^n \tag{5.10}$$

$$x_0 \quad \longmapsto \quad \Phi_{t_0}^{t_1}(x_0) = x_0 + \int_{t_0}^{t_1} u(x(t_1),t)\mathrm{d}t = x(t_1;t_0,x_0). \tag{5.11}$$

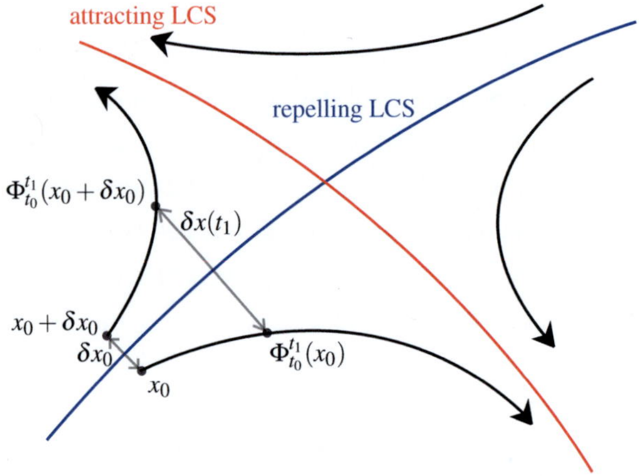

Figure 5.5: Schematic sketch of the evolution of the distance between two particles, δx_0, (blue) repelled by an LCS and (red) attracted by an LCS. Sketch adapted from Kaiser (2014).

In order to measure the stretching of the initial infinitesimal distance δx_0, the Cauchy-Green deformation tensor $\mathbf{C}$ is calculated based on the previously defined flow map

$$\mathbf{C} = (\nabla\Phi_{t_0}^{t_1})^{\mathrm{T}}\nabla\Phi_{t_0}^{t_1}. \tag{5.12}$$

Information on the folding and stretching within the flow field is obtained by determining the eigenvalues of the positive definite Cauchy-Green tensor. The largest eigenvalue λ_{max} corresponds to the maximum particle separation and the corresponding eigenvector gives the stretching direction. The FTLE $\sigma_{t_0}^{t_1}$ itself is obtained by scaling λ_{max}

$$\sigma_{t_0}^{t_1} = \frac{1}{|T_{int}|} \ln \sqrt{\lambda_{max}}. \tag{5.13}$$

Hyperbolic LCS are now defined as ridges consisting of the maximum FTLE values as these form the planes of the highest separation rate. Following Schindler et al. [81], λ_{max} already contains all the needed information for visualising the desired LCS. As the natural logarithm and the square root are monotone functions, they flatten the input parameter. Therefore, the differences between LCS of alternate strengths become less dominant. Kaiser (2014) suggests that especially in highly complex flows, e.g. the heart flow, it might be beneficial to highlight only the strongest LCS and therefore skip parts of the applied scaling in Equation (5.13).

The following degrees of freedom influence the resulting FTLE field:

interpolation method

For the flow map evaluation the underlying discrete velocity data has to be interpolated. The data presented in this work is based on linear interpolation to keep computational costs low.

integration time

LCS that appear and vanish during the integration time might not be detected, as only the separation between the particle starting point and the final position determine the FTLE value. However, Shadden et al. [89] and Kaiser (2014) state that with longer integration times more LCS are revealed. The more LCS are detected the more difficult is the interpretation of the results.

VP

The number of discrete Eulerian velocity points (VP) determines the size of the underlying velocity mesh for which the LCS are to be extracted. VP itself is defined with respect to a characteristic length of the flow field.

PP

The particle mesh consists of the chosen number of particle points (*PP*) that shall be tracked when the flow map is generated. Thus, the amount of *PP* determines the number of calculated FTLE values. *PP* is defined with respect to the same characteristic length as VP.

TP

When the time-dependent velocity field is stored, it has to be decided how many time points (TP) per characteristic time interval are needed for the computation of the FTLE field.

The central scientific question determines the duration of the integration time T_{int}. In the example of the periodic heart flow an integration time equal to one heart beat uncovers which volume portions enter or leave the heart during the regarded beat. This information serves as basis for the determination of particle residence times.

A correctly determined FTLE field is necessary for a reliable LCS detection that provides meaningful information. Up to now, it is not clear how to choose the different resolutions, i.e. the spatial and temporal resolution of the underlying velocity field (VP and TP) and the spatial resolution of the tracked particles (*PP*). With finer resolutions the costs for the mathematical procedure and especially the necessary memory increase. Therefore, the objective is to determine the ideal resolutions for the heart flow examination. An ideal resolution is as coarse as possible and as fine as necessary.

To study the specific influence of VP, *PP* and TP and to develop and test evaluation criteria, the FTLE is applied to the double gyre flow introduced in Chapter 5.1. Here, a characteristic length, L_c, is defined equal to the diameter of the two vortices which is restricted by the height of the flow domain (compare Figure 5.6). As the objective is to define a consistent resolution for different flow cases, the two spatial resolutions VP and PP are defined based on how many velocity or particle points are distributed along the characteristic length. Therefore, increasing values yield finer resolutions. Hereby, the resolution of the two meshes are independent from each other. Only equidistant meshes are regarded in the current investigation. In Figure 5.6 the resolution of the velocity mesh on the left hand side is $VP = 3$, marked with crosses along L_c, and the resolution of the particle mesh on the right hand side is $PP = 5$, marked with circles along L_c. Each velocity information or particle build a corner in the respective mesh. The two spatial resolutions are independent of each other and can be chosen separately.

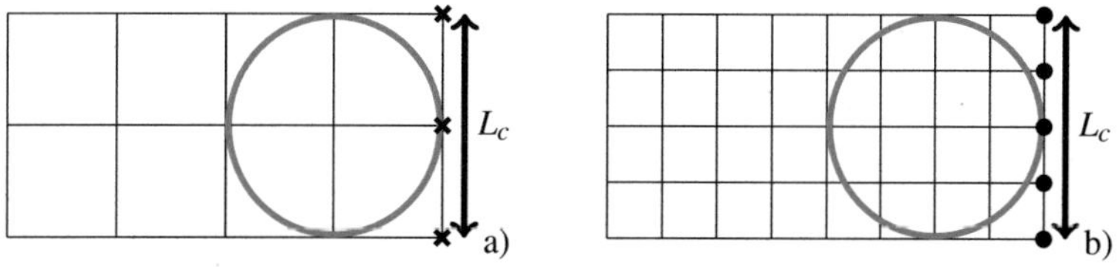

Figure 5.6: Schematic representation of a) the underlying velocity mesh with $VP = 3$ (crosses) and b) the underlying particle distribution with $PP = 5$ (circles).

In accordance with the spatial resolutions, the temporal resolution of the underlying velocity field is defined with respect to a characteristic time. In the cases of the double gyre and the heart flow, a characteristic time is represented by the length of one period. Throughout the following sections the resolutions VP, PP and TP are varied for the double gyre flow. More detailed information about the examinations summarised in the following subsections are provided by Gollub (2015) and Brakhage (2016). Equivalent evaluations based on the 2D von Kármán vortex street are summarised in Appendix A.2. Supplementary investigations are reported by Gollub (2015) who investigates additionally a piston vortex. Those 3D results confirm the findings for the 2D fields presented here.

5.2.1 Spatial Resolution of the Particle Tracking

Between two particles only one LCS can be detected. As such, some LCS and important flow characteristics are not found if *PP* is too low. Literature includes some methods to find good approximations of LCS even with low particle numbers [28, 79, 88]. One possibility is to start with a coarse mesh and refine regions where high separation rates are detected. However, in order to understand the influence of the particle mesh resolution and to find a general guideline for the needed number of tracked particles, an equidistant particle distribution is used.

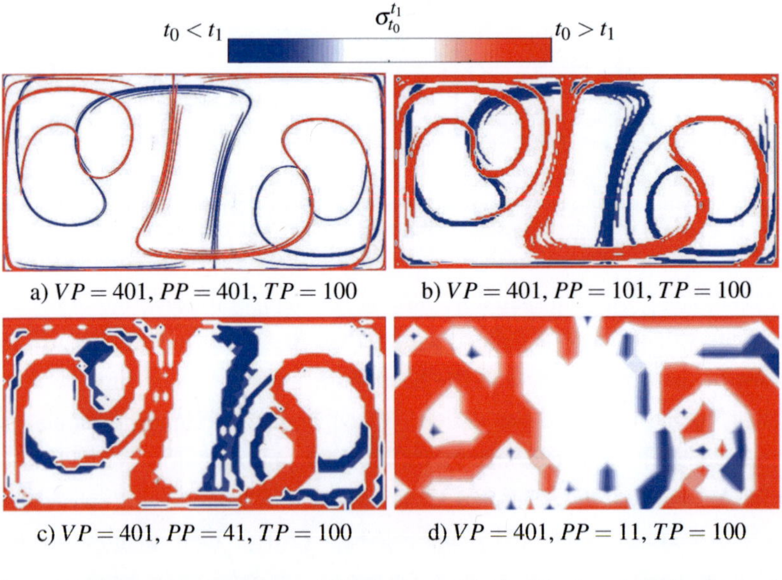

a) $VP = 401, PP = 401, TP = 100$ b) $VP = 401, PP = 101, TP = 100$

c) $VP = 401, PP = 41, TP = 100$ d) $VP = 401, PP = 11, TP = 100$

Figure 5.7: Ridges of the (blue) forward FTLE value and the (red) backward FTLE value for the double gyre flow with $T_{int} = 15\,\text{s}$. VP and TP are constant. The resolution of PP decreases from a) to d).

Figure 5.7 a) shows a forward FTLE (blue) and a backward FTLE (red) of the double gyre flow with $VP = 401$, $PP = 401$ and $TP = 100$. The integration time is $T_{int} = 15\,\text{s}$, which covers 1.5 periods of the flow. According to Gollub (2015) these resolutions are finer than necessary for appropriate LCS detection. Only the FTLE values higher than 60% of the maximum value are shown and scaled by the respective maximum of the field. In doing so, FTLE ridges are extracted and thus LCS are visualised. Throughout Figure 5.7 b), c) and d), VP and TP are kept constant and PP decreases. Thereby, the ridges of the FTLE value remain at the same location but loose their sharpness in comparison to the finest resolution.

The mathematical definition of the FTLE value is based on an infinitesimal particle distance in the starting position. This value is never reached in the numerical calculation and therefore the determined values never reach the analytical ones [87]. The maximum FTLE value depends on the numerical scheme of the Cauchy-Green tensor calculation and decreases with a decreasing PP resolution. This is mathematically shown for the double gyre by Kaiser (2014).

In general, the maximum particle separation results if two infinitesimal close pathlines reach the maximum possible distance at the end of the integration time. As a consequence, the difference between the two corresponding flow maps, $\delta\Phi_{t_0}^{t_1}$, is equal to the size of the domain bounding box. In case of the double gyre flow, this is

$$\delta\Phi_{t_0}^{t_1} = \begin{pmatrix} 2 \\ 1 \end{pmatrix}. \tag{5.14}$$

Assuming an equidistant grid, where the grid spacing is $\Delta x = \Delta y = const$, the trace of $\mathbf{C}$ is approximated using central differences:

$$\begin{aligned}
\mathrm{tr}(\mathbf{C}) &= \left(\frac{\delta\Phi_{t_0,x}^{t_1}}{2\Delta x}\right)^2 + \left(\frac{\delta\Phi_{t_0,y}^{t_1}}{2\Delta x}\right)^2 + \left(\frac{\delta\Phi_{t_0,x}^{t_1}}{2\Delta y}\right)^2 + \left(\frac{\delta\Phi_{t_0,y}^{t_1}}{2\Delta y}\right)^2 \\
&= \frac{5}{2}\frac{1}{(\Delta x)^2}. \qquad (5.15)
\end{aligned}$$

In 2D, the maximum eigenvalue, λ_{max}, of the Cauchy-Green Tensor, $\mathbf{C}$, is expressed via

$$\lambda_{max}(\mathbf{C}) = \frac{1}{2}\left(\mathrm{tr}(\mathbf{C}) + \sqrt{(\mathrm{tr}(\mathbf{C}))^2 - 4\det(\mathbf{C})}\right) = \frac{5}{2}\frac{1}{(\Delta x)^2} \approx PP^2. \qquad (5.16)$$

Equation (5.16) shows that the FTLE value depends on the grid spacing of *PP*. It increases with increasing resolution. This fact has to be kept in mind when FTLE fields shall be quantitatively compared. These observations lead to the question of how many particles must be seeded into the flow to obtain a sharp and meaningful LCS. An estimation has been presented for judging the resultant FTLE resolution [SSKK14]. The findings are shortly presented in the following.

As two particle meshes with different resolutions cannot be compared pointwise, the sum of all FTLE values, $\sum \sigma_i$, is taken for comparison. The evolution of the sum, shown in Figure 5.8, reflects not only the increasing mean FTLE value with increasing *PP*, but also the increasing number of FTLE values with increasing *PP*. In loglog scale the sum correlates with the particle refinement rate shown by the light-grey dashed line with inclination 2 : 1. This conclusion is valid for fields where the Euclidean norm of the Jacobian is restricted by

$$\left\| \frac{\mathrm{d}\Phi_{t_0}^{t_1}}{\mathrm{d}x} \right\| \leq \mathrm{e}^{k_1|t_1 - t_0|}, \qquad (5.17)$$

with $k_1 = const$ [89]. If the underlying velocity field is Lipschitz continuous, this condition holds true for all times t_1. The sum of all FTLE values can be determined by multiplying the mean FTLE value $\bar{\sigma}$ and the total number of particles N. For the double gyre the sum is then expressed by

$$\sum_{i=1..N} \sigma_i = \bar{\sigma}N = \bar{\sigma}(2PP^2 - PP). \tag{5.18}$$

Here, the characteristic length scale is chosen to be equal to the domain height which is half of the domain width. The total number of particles is then determined via $2PP^2$, corresponding to the particles in the two domain halves, and a correction of $-PP$. Without the correction, particles distributed along the centreline are counted twice.

The sum of FTLE values in the finest tested resolution, $\max\left(\sum \sigma_i\right) = \lim_{N \to \infty} \sum \sigma_i$, provides an ideal mean value that serves as comparison with lower resolutions. This ideal value is used to determine the theoretical sum, $\sum \sigma_{i,theor}$, that would result if the resolution of PP was fine enough. It can therefore be used for direct comparison with the actual value. A proof of the obtained result uses an interpolation of the calculated FTLE field onto the finest reference resolution. The resultant sum, $\sum \sigma_{i,interp}$, is included in Figure 5.8. It shows that, for a constant PP, the sum and therefore the mean value of the FTLE field is limited by a constant and satisfies Equation (5.17).

As a first estimate, a discrepancy of 3 % between the ideal sum and the actual sum is arbitrarily chosen, which results for the double gyre in $PP \geq 52$ as sufficient resolution for all tested VP. Inspecting the results visually, this finding is confirmed. The result is independent of the chosen characteristic length and the sum criterion holds true for multiple tested flow scenarios (see Appendix A.2). As such, it is not limited to cases with a known vortex diameter.

The practical application should start with a coarse resolution and subsequently compare the sum with the next finer resolution [SGK+15]. Figure 5.9 shows the resulting deviation, ε, for the comparison with a reference field and the comparison with the finer neighbouring field. Both approaches overlap for $PP \geq 40$.

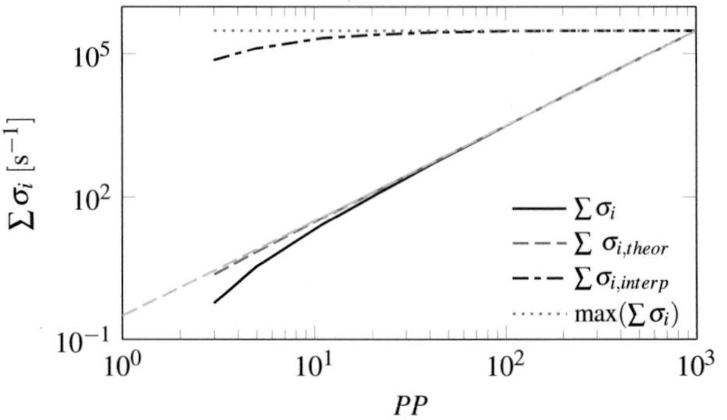

Figure 5.8: The sum of all FTLE values, obtained from forward integration with $VP = 1001$ for varying PP, is compared to interpolated and theoretical values.

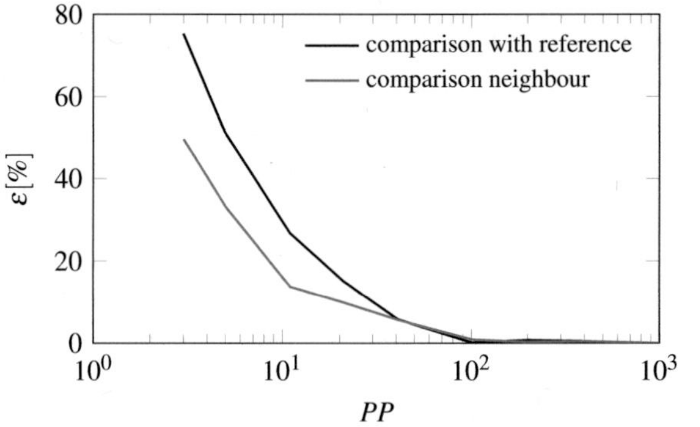

Figure 5.9: Resulting error of the mean FTLE value for varying PP with respect to either the finest reference solution or the next finer neighbouring solution.

The threshold leading to a sufficient resolution applicable in all different kinds of cases has still to be found. Concerning this matter, Gollub (2015) highlights that the necessary resolution of PP strongly depends on the chosen integration time. Obviously, an increase of the integration time has to be accompanied by increasing *PP* to ensure the detection of developing LCS over time.

5.2.2 Spatial Resolution of the Underlying Velocity Data

The mesh resolution of CFD or number of pixels recorded in an experimental set-up determine the number and resolution of detected flow field features. Alike other post-processing tools, the FTLE is dependent on the information available within the underlying velocity field. If the resolution of the Eulerian data is low, important characteristics might be undetectable. Comparable with a mesh independence study, VP is varied in the following to determine its influence on the FTLE results.

In theory, the underlying velocity field determined through CFD could be altered in two ways, either deleting existing velocity points in the field or recalculating the field with a different resolution. The latter might change the characteristics of the flow itself and the FTLE field. A differentiation where discrepancies in the FTLE originate from is not possible. Thus, the approach of manipulating an existing flow field is chosen.

Figure 5.10 a) shows the forward FTLE (blue) and the backward FTLE (red) of the double gyre flow with $VP = 41$, $PP = 401$ and $TP = 100$. Although $PP \geq 52$ is determined to be a sufficient particle resolution, a higher number is chosen to ensure that no reciprocal effects come into play. Again, only the FTLE values higher than 60% of the maximum are shown and scaled by the respective maximum value. Throughout Figure 5.10 b), c) and d) *PP* and TP are kept constant and VP decreases. Thereby, the ridges of the FTLE field remain sharp but alter their shape and position in comparison to the finest resolution.

A local point by point comparison of the results with different VP is possible because *PP* remains constant throughout this examination and equals the number of calculated FTLE values [SGK+15]. As such, for every particle p, the difference between its FTLE value and the FTLE value of the reference configuration is calculated. To obtain a local relative error $\varepsilon(p)$, the subtraction is scaled by the sum of the corresponding FTLE values. Thereby, the whole field information is equally taken into account, no matter if the particle is located on an FTLE ridge or within a region of small FTLE values. The resultant $\varepsilon(p)$ is always within the interval $[0,1]$:

$$\varepsilon(p) = \frac{|\sigma_p| - |\sigma_{ref}|}{\sigma_p + \sigma_{ref}}. \tag{5.19}$$

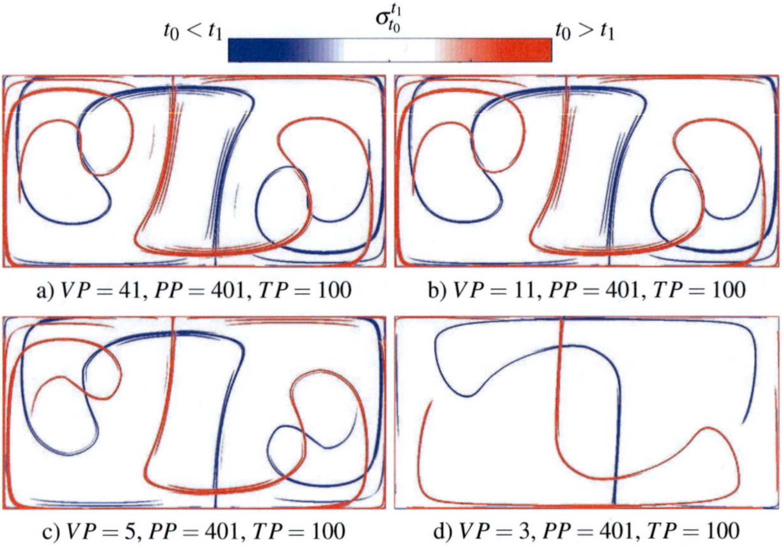

Figure 5.10: Ridges of the (blue) forward FTLE value and the (red) backward FTLE value for the double gyre flow with $T_{int} = 15\,\mathrm{s}$. PP and TP are constant. The resolution of VP decreases from a) to d).

Comparing the mean and the median of the relative error reveals that the distribution of the local relative error includes a significant number of outliers, which can be filtered if the median is applied. These observations are confirmed by visual inspection of the results. Therefore, the median,

$$\hat{\varepsilon} = \begin{cases} \varepsilon(p)_{\frac{N+1}{2}} & \text{if } N \text{ is odd} \\ \frac{1}{2}\left(\varepsilon(p)_{\frac{N}{2}} + \varepsilon(p)_{\frac{N+1}{2}}\right) & \text{if } N \text{ is even} \end{cases}, \tag{5.20}$$

is chosen as global measure for comparison of two configurations, with N being the amount of particles.

Figure 5.11 shows the slope of the global relative error, $\hat{\varepsilon}$, for varying VP at different constant resolutions of PP [SGK$^+$15]. Following the procedure of the sum criterion in the previous section, a discrepancy of 3% is exemplary chosen as acceptance threshold. For the double gyre, this leads to $VP \geq 10$ being sufficiently resolved to obtain correctly positioned LCS. This result is confirmed by visual inspection of the FTLE fields. This finding correlates well with the practices in CFD, where ten cells are known to be advisable for a proper reproduction of flow structures.

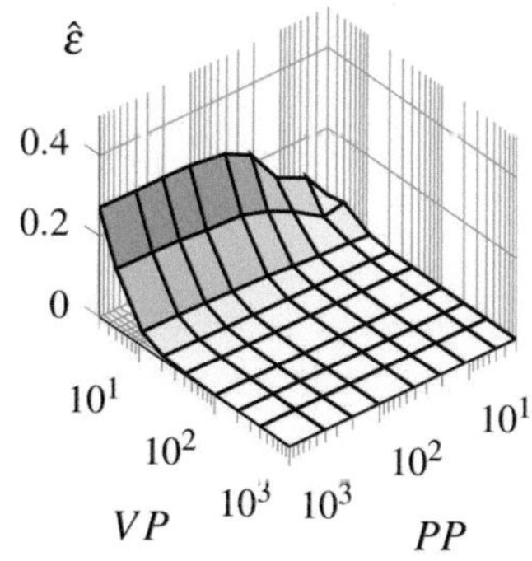

Figure 5.11: The relative error obtained from forward integration with varying VP and PP.

For a coarse resolution of VP, an increasing number of PP leads to a rising relative error (compare Figure 5.11) due to two accompanying effects. Firstly, small FTLE values are stronger affected by the numerical imprecision than large FTLE value. The amount of small FTLE values is significantly larger, since large FTLE values are only found on the ridges of the FTLE field. In contrast to the sum criterion, the relative error uses a local value comparison and is thus directly affected by the local numerical imprecision which grows with the number of particles. This effect is reduced with an increasing number of VP which increases the accuracy of the determined particle paths. Secondly, the resulting sharpening of the LCS leads to steeper spatial gradients within the FTLE field. Therefore, an increasing particle resolution rises the sensitivity of the relative error on local changes in the field. If local changes are introduced by measurement discrepancies, e.g. originating from faulty repositioning of the camera between two consecutive measurements, the relative error reports insufficient velocity resolution. That is why the use of this method is only recommended, if the underlying data is reproducible with high confidence.

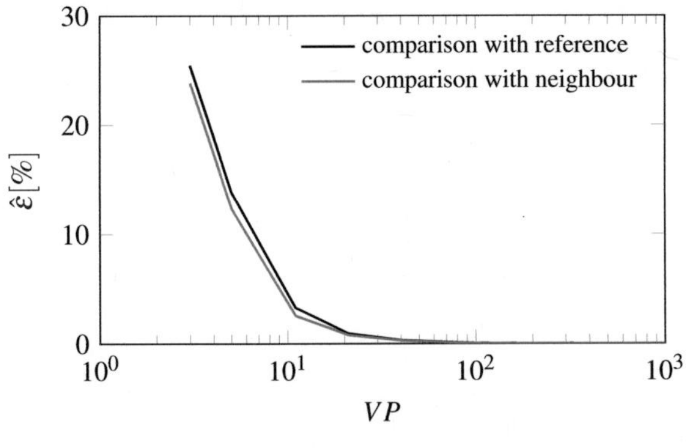

Figure 5.12: Resulting global relative error comparing the local FTLE value to either the finest reference solution or the finer neighbouring solution.

The practical application should start with a coarse resolution and subsequently compare the sum with the finer neighbouring resolution [SGK$^+$15].

Figure 5.12 shows the resulting deviation for the comparison with a reference field and the comparison with the finer neighbouring field. Both approaches overlap for $VP \geq 20$ and suggest a sufficient resolution of $VP \geq 10$. This result is confirmed by visual inspection. The evaluation of the relative error for the von Kármán vortex street yields the same result (see Appendix A.2).

5.2.3 Temporal Resolution of the Underlying Velocity Data

The last resolution that is to be tested is the temporal resolution of the underlying velocity field. Alike the spatial resolution, the number of available time points per period TP determines whether all important characteristics of the flow can be reliably detected.

Figure 5.13 a) shows the forward FTLE (blue) and the backward FTLE (red) of the double gyre flow with $VP = 401$, $PP = 401$ and $TP = 10$. Choosing the respective spatial resolutions of VP and PP ensures that no reciprocal effects come into play. Again, only the FTLE values higher than 60% of the maximum are shown and scaled by the respective maximum value. Throughout Figure 5.13 b), c) and d) VP and PP are kept constant and TP decreases. Thereby, the ridges of the FTLE field remain sharp but alter their shape and position in comparison to the finest resolution. It is worth noting that a $TP = 2$ (compare Figure 5.13) results in two identical flow fields per period, where the middle axis between the two vortices is located in the centre of the x-axis. As such, the underlying velocity data becomes steady and the centreline forms the only separatrix. The LCS along the bounding box wall purely originate from wall shear effects.

In order to determine how many TP provide a reasonable resolution, Brakhage (2016) applies the sum of all FTLE values and the relative error to the double gyre flow with varying time resolution. His method is adapted in the following. As in the previous sections, the current configuration is either compared to the finest reference resolution or to the finer neighbouring resolution. Further, the steps in which TP increases are chosen to be fine, in steps of $0.01TP$

or coarse, ongoing doubled. The results are shown in Figure 5.14 for the sum criterion and Figure 5.15 for the relative error criterion. Application of the sum criterion shows overall smaller errors compared to the relative error. This is expected, because the influence of a changing TP is comparable to the influence of a changing VP, where the local displacement is more affected than the quantitative numbers. Further, two FTLE fields can be very different in appearance but have the same sum.

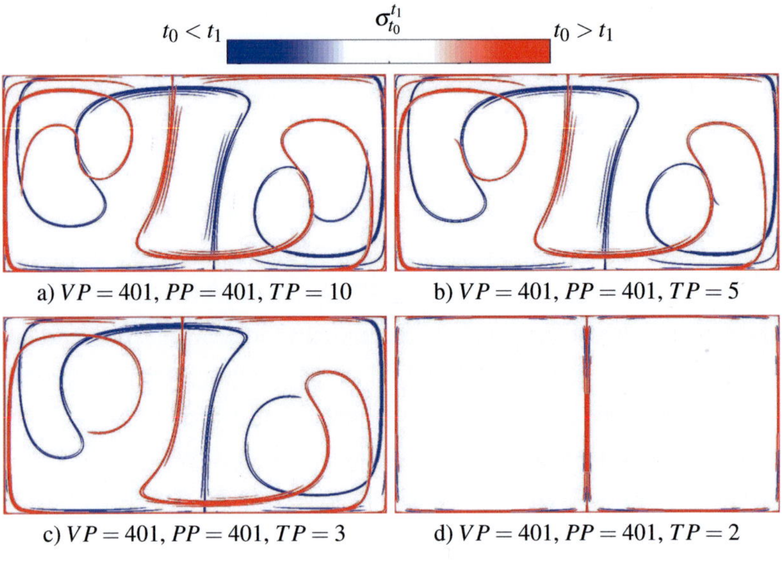

Figure 5.13: Ridges of the (blue) forward FTLE value and the (red) backward FTLE value for the double gyre flow with $T_{int} = 15$s. PP and VP are constant. The resolution of TP decreases from a) to d).

All strategies result in three distinguishable zones that can be associated to the nature of the underlying velocity field:

quasi Eulerian – Area I: $TP < 10^0$

For low numbers of TP, the particle paths are close or even equal to the streamlines of the flow field. Choosing the method of coarse TP

steps yields a constant error, as the periodicity of the velocity field in combination with the chosen TP yields a steady flow. Thus, the FTLE field is constant. For fine TP steps, a fluctuation appears in the error criteria caused by the appearance of a beat frequency. Here, some values of TP result in velocity field information slightly shifted in comparison to half periods. Care has to be taken, when the neighbouring field is chosen for comparison. In the quasi Eulerian regime, it often leads to errors close to zero and therefore the FTLE might be wrongly assessed as correct.

transitioning from Eulerian to Lagrangian – Area II: $10^0 < TP < 10^1$

In the transition zone, the underlying velocity develops from quasi steady to an approximation of the unsteady physical analytical field. This leads first to a rising error in all approaches, when the time-dependency becomes more dominant and the pathlines noticeably diverge from the streamlines. The error decreases as soon as the velocity field approaches a well resolved unsteady flow field and the determined pathlines approximate the analytical ones.

Lagrangian – Area III: $10^1 < TP$

For $TP > 10^1$, more than ten velocity fields are available per period. Here, the development of the error criteria suggests that a good approximation of the continuous analytical function is reached. This hypothesis is confirmed by visual inspection of the FTLE fields. In case of the double gyre, an error threshold of 3% results in a too low TP resolution, whereas a threshold of 1% fits the detected bound ($TP \geq 11$).

The described curve progressions confirm the findings of Kaiser et al. [46]. The application of the introduced error criteria to the von Kármán vortex street shows that they are not limited to internal closed domains. The resulting error progressions are shown in Appendix A.2.

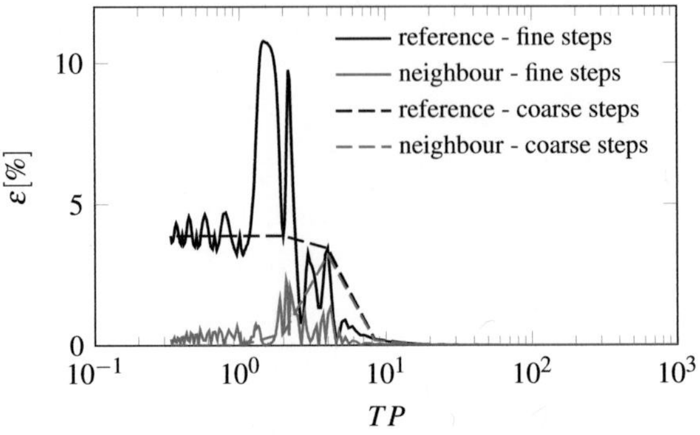

Figure 5.14: Resulting error of the sum criterion compared to either the finest reference solution or the finer neighbouring solution. TP is altered in coarse steps, ongoing doubled, or fine steps of $0.01TP$.

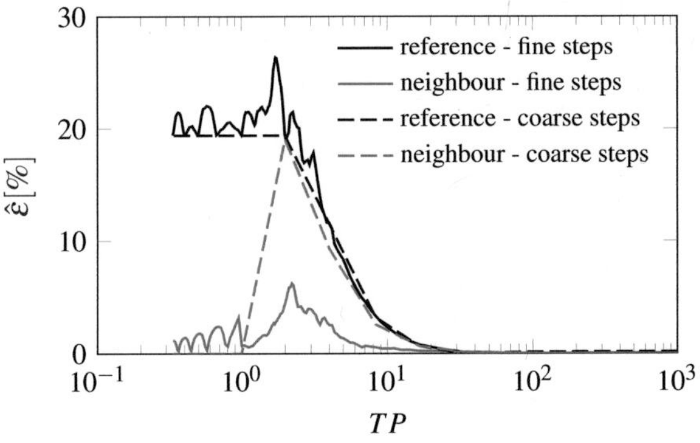

Figure 5.15: Global relative error comparing the local FTLE value to either the finest reference solution or the finer neighbouring solution. TP is altered in coarse steps, ongoing doubled, or fine steps of $0.01TP$.

5.2.4 Superposition of Spatial and Temporal Resolution

In practical application, the underlying flow characteristics are often unknown. Up to now, it is not possible to judge whether the combination of the independently detected resolutions (*PP*, *VP* and *TP*) still yields a good estimate. The question arises, how well the identified criteria react to superimposed influences of the resolutions. Therefore, an error ε_{max} that is equal to the maximum of the mean FTLE error and the global relative error is introduced:

$$\varepsilon_{max} = \max(\varepsilon, \hat{\varepsilon}). \tag{5.21}$$

This combined error allows a comparison of all present influences. It is first shown for a combined variation of the spatial resolutions, *PP* and *VP* (see Figure 5.16). Due to the symmetry of the double gyre flow, forward and backward FTLE fields are reflections of each other. Thus, the resulting error maps are equal.

Comparing the progressions of lines in Figure 5.16 along different constant *PP* or *VP* to each other shows that their shape is not remarkably altered with the resolution of the respective constant. Coarse resolution of one quantity raises and flattens the overall error curve of the other. This effect is visible as soon as the respective resolution reaches the critical resolution detected before. Superimposing the effects of altering *PP* and *VP* has little effect on the resulting error, as the resolution of the FTLE field and the positioning of the FTLE ridges are independent of each other.

Two lines are added to the error plots. They indicate the chosen 3% error bound of the criteria. The point where the threshold lines meet marks the point of minimum required resolution. At the same time, the point indicates the minimum required computational effort for obtaining accurate results.

Figure 5.17 additionally includes the variation of the temporal resolution. Exemplary slices are chosen for the visualisation of the 3D error field. The positioning of the LCS is now influenced by the temporal and the spatial resolution. Thus, the relative error dominates over the error of the mean FTLE value. The interaction of temporal and both spatial resolutions is similar to the observed effects when combining only the spatial resolutions (VP and PP). A coarsening of TP raises the error progressions of both criteria to higher levels. However, it affects the relative error to a greater extent. Having in mind that the spatial and temporal resolution of the underlying velocity field (VP and TP respectively) both affect the positioning of the LCS, it is clear that the effect is enhanced if both resolutions are coarsened.

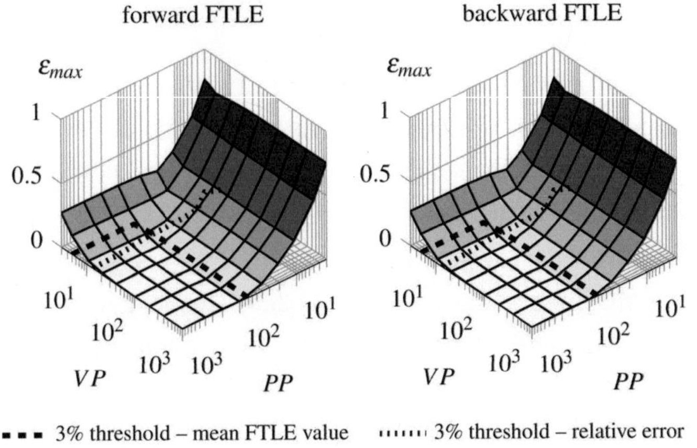

Figure 5.16: Double gyre: Combined global relative error and mean FTLE error for varying PP and VP at $TP = 100$. The comparison is performed with the finest reference solution.

Unfortunately, a precise distinction whether an error in LCS positioning originates in the spatial or temporal resolution is not possible. Whether an error originates in the particle seeding can always be verified by visual inspection of the resulting field sharpness. Nonetheless, a careful variation of all parameters is recommended in practical application.

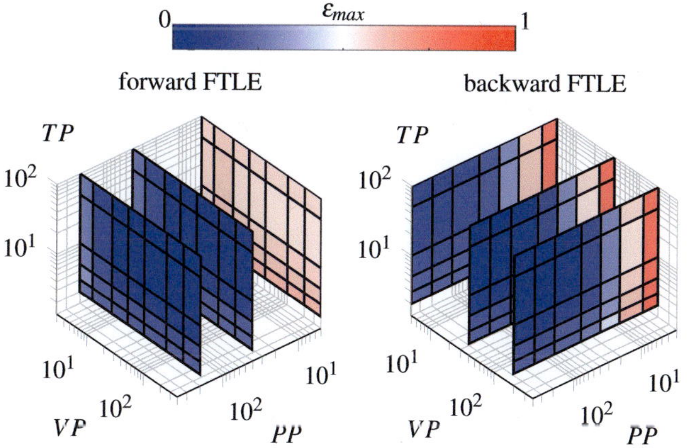

Figure 5.17: Double gyre: Combined global relative error and mean FTLE error for varying PP, VP and TP. The comparison is performed with the finest reference solution.

5.2.5 Evaluation of Error Influences

The basis velocity data used for FTLE calculations are discrete in space (either 2D or 3D) and time. When a particle path is determined via integration, the field information has to be interpolated at the current particle position. In general multiple options are available, e.g. first-order linear or third-order polynomial [58]. The examples shown in this work are determined using linear interpolation in order to minimise the necessary random access memory. However, a high-order interpolation cannot compensate insufficient field resolutions [SGK⁺15]. Once information is lost in the underlying data, the vortex detection methods cannot increase the accuracy.

Nonetheless, small errors in the interpolation of the particle position (spatial as well as temporal) can sum up over time and produce significant errors in the final result [87]. Different trials show that the LCS is fortunately robust in terms of the integrated error influences [36, 70, 90]. Especially the most repelling and attracting ridges are resistant against local temporal errors, i.e. temporary velocity peaks [35].

The influence of a persistent error in the velocity fields, i.e. measurement noise, is evaluated by Olcay et al. [70] and Brakhage (2016). Both come to the conclusion that the LCS position is on average not affected.

Kaiser (2014) chooses the ode45 solver [58] to perform the integration of the pathlines as it is robust, fast and accurate. Although the pathline calculation is not efficient in stiff problems, it is still accurate. Thus, the integration process itself does not introduce critical errors.

In contrast to the double gyre, the human heart has open boundaries, where fluid particles can pass through. If a particle leaves the computational domain, its velocity has to be extrapolated as accurately as possible to minimise resulting errors in the FTLE calculation (compare Kaiser (2014)).

5.3 Combination of the Vortex Detection Methods

The particular manner of FTLE implementation used in this work yields two types of LCS: hyperbolic LCS and shear induced LCS . In general, the classical FTLE measures the separation rate of flow particles independent of the separation direction. Thereby, shear induced separation where the particle paths can be parallel to each other, e.g. found in boundary layers, is detected as well as normal repulsion of attraction, i.e. hyperbolic LCS. Since regions of high shear can affect the blood particles, their identification is no drawback.

A region in the double gyre flow where shear separates particles is the central axis between the vortices. The velocity vectors between the core of one vortex and the centre line are oriented parallel. Further, flow rotation is not the Q dominating component in proximity to the flow stagnation points at the top and the bottom of the central axis (compare Figure 5.3). As seen previously in Section 5.1, shear forces acting on a fluid element induce a combination of pure strain and rotation. If this rotation is persistent over time, the axis of the rate-of-strain tensor rotate over time. In order to obtain a clear separation between local rotation and local strain, the Q-criterion can be modified following Tabor and Klapper [95] as

$$Q' = \frac{1}{2}((\| \Omega_{ij} - \Omega'_{ij} \|)^2 - (\| S_{ij} \|)^2), \tag{5.22}$$

where Ω'_{ij} represents the rotation rate of the strain axes. Then, $Q' < 0$ identifies local strain. However, the implementation of Ω'_{ij} for general application is costly as it involve Lagrangian tracking of the strain axes. Tabor and Klapper [95] further state that the Q-criterion as defined in Equation (5.6) clearly identifies rotation dominated fluid motion, while $Q > 0$ identifies strain dominated motion with a tendency for local stretching.

Figure 5.18 superimposes a forward and a backward LCS for the double with the Q-criterion at two different time point. The integration time for the LCS generation is chosen to be a half period. Thereby, the interpretation is simplified. The visualisation shows, how the Q-criterion gives insights into the flow effects that lead to particle separation. Close to the stagnation points, the flow strain pushes the particles apart, while the influence of flow rotation increases with an increasing distance from the wall.

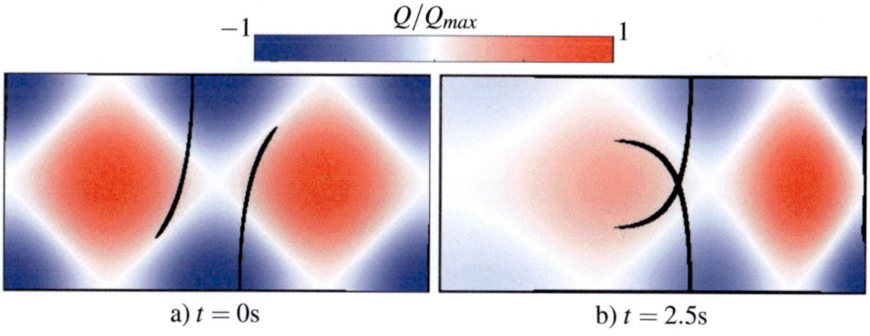

Figure 5.18: Double gyre: Q-criterion superimposed by backward and forward LCS determined with an integration time of $T_{int} = 5$ s.

The observed capacities of the two vortex detection methods enable in combination the extraction of various flow information particular important for the blood flow: vortex generation and propagation, regions of dominating strain, cause-effect relations, mixing processes and particle residence times. All these quantities are helpful for determination of a patient's health status.

A meaningful data extraction for comparison of different heart flow cases becomes possible with the choice of appropriate vortex detection methods and the development of the criteria to determine the proper resolutions. Thus, the Q-criterion and the FTLE are applied to the flow fields that result in the LV from different MV models in the following chapter.

6 Numerical Investigation of an Idealised Left Ventricle

This chapter presents an investigation of two different MV models included in an idealised LV, in order to evaluate their influences on vortex generation and development in the LV. Hereby, a simple and a complex model are chosen to enable drawing conclusions about valid simplifications in the MV geometry.

The LV test geometry is extracted from magnetic resonance imaging (MRI) data of a healthy human [49] and can be seen in Figure 6.1. The aorta and the pulmonary veins are represented by elongated straight tubes. Thereby, these boundaries do not significantly influence the flow inside of the ventricle and backflow across inlet or outlet is prevented. Further, the number of pulmonary veins is reduced from four to two, whereby computational costs are reduced. It was shown that the reduction does not influence the flow in the ventricle [92].

In all simulations presented in this work, the volumetric change of the ventricular wall generates the pumping force that drives the flow. Therefore, the pressure is prescribed at the inlets (pulmonary veins) and the outlet (aorta) by means of a Dirichlet boundary condition. OpenFOAM-1.6-ext is a finite volume solver that solves the NSE (2.5) in a flux-based formulation. The flux boundary conditions at inlets and outlet are Neumann boundary conditions, such that the volume flux can adjust automatically to the generated volume change. This means that the velocity is determined based on the resultant fluxes. All geometry walls have a no-slip condition for the flux and a gradient-free condition for the pressure. Thus, every boundary is associated with a Dirichlet and a Neumann condition so that the system of equations is fully determined. Details on solver settings have been discussed in Chapter 3 and are listed in Appendix A.1.

Further model simplifications include a steady LA, because the flow within the LV is in the focus of the examination. The LV movement is prescribed by an analytical function that determines the displacement of the boundary points, Δx_i, in dependency of their current position on the x-axis and the length of the ventricle, L_V, measured from the apex to the MV annulus. A reference point, $(0.04\,\text{m}, -0.005\,\text{m}, 0.01\,\text{m})$, is located in the LV centre such that each boundary point moves along the vector that connects it with the centre. Thereby, folding of the geometry is prevented. The LV reaches an end diastolic volume of 186 ml and an ejection fraction of

$$EF = \frac{V_{dia} - V_{sys}}{V_{dia}} = \frac{V_{stroke}}{V_{dia}} = 23\,\%, \tag{6.1}$$

which gives the ratio of stroke volume to the end diastolic volume. These values are chosen in close proximity to other validation studies conducted with the same geometry [48, 92].

$$x_{rel} = x - x_{min} - \tfrac{1}{3}L_V \tag{6.2}$$

$$\varphi = \begin{cases} 0, & x_{rel} < 0 \\ 3\frac{x_{rel}}{L_V}, & x_{rel} < \frac{1}{3}L_V \\ \frac{3}{2} - \frac{3}{2}\frac{x_{rel}}{L_V}, & x_{rel} > \frac{1}{3}L_V \end{cases} \tag{6.3}$$

$$x_i = \begin{pmatrix} x - 0.04 \\ y + 0.005 \\ z - 0.01 \end{pmatrix} \tag{6.4}$$

$$\Delta x_i = 0.028\varphi \sin(2\pi t)\frac{x_i}{\|x_i\|} \tag{6.5}$$

The flow is considered to be laminar and incompressible (compare Chapter 4). Based on the MV diameter, $d_{MV} = 15\,\text{mm}$, and a kinematic viscosity of $\nu = 3.8 \cdot 10^{-6}\text{m}^2\,\text{s}^{-1}$ [22], the maximum Reynolds number reached is $\text{Re} = 2760$. The Womersley number lies in the physiological range, with $\text{Wo} = 19.29$, and the Strouhal number is low enough to be connected to an unhealthy status, with $\text{St} = 0.02$, which is expected remembering the resultant ejection fraction. According to the mesh independence study carried out by Spiegel [92], the mesh should consist of a minimum of 100,000 cells in an ALE framework. Because ALE formulation and IBM are both used, a finer mesh of 200,000 cells is used that is expected to conserve the boundary of the immersed geometry. Further, the amount of cells constitutes the necessary VP resolution for the extraction of LCS in the post-processing. The simulations start with an initial time step of $\Delta t_0 = 0.001\,\text{s}$. Afterwards, the time stepping is adjusted automatically to satisfy $CFL = 0.7$. At the initialisation of the solver the fluid is at rest. The pressure-volume diagram shows that the flow results reach a periodic state after five consecutive heart beats.

In the following section an overview of the literature on available MV models is given. Based on the findings, two models are chosen and implemented into the LV geometry in order to evaluate their influences on vortex generation and development in the LV.

6.1 Available Mitral Valve Models

Bakar (2015) gives an overview over the research carried out on the mitral valve that involves fluid flow around the leaflets. She divides the different model approaches into five categories and evaluates them as follows:

diode type MV model

The valve's closing and opening is mimicked by blocking or allowing the fluid to pass through the valve plane [53, 54, 55, 77, 85, 86, 102, 104, 109, 110]. Besides the blocking, the fluid is not affected by the valve model.

From all available MV models, this is the easiest and fastest approach. Some examples in the literature show that this model is not capable to capture the physiological flow conditions in the LV in a satisfying manner [85, 86].

planar MV model

This more complex diode type model is based on imaging techniques and mimics the effective opening area of the MV through gradual opening of the valve plane area [7, 8, 21, 49, 65, 66, 67, 68, 80]. Therefore, the MV plane is blocked during the systole and opened by varying the size of the mitral orifice. In general, no physical wall movement is considered. The computational costs are comparable to the previous model and it was shown that this approach yields the expected flow characteristics [48, 92]. To the author's knowledge, direct comparison to a more physiological model has not been done so far.

geometry-prescribed MV model

While the valve leaflets are inserted into the fluid flow, the mechanics of the valve are not determined. Instead, the motion of the leaflets is prescribed according to measurements or simplified functions [5, 8, 15, 60, 86, 103]. The wall motion can be realised using ALE or IBM (see Chapter 2.3). The model can reach different levels of complexity depending on how accurate the shape and the motion shall be modelled. The level of complexity is directly linked to the computational costs.

FSI MV model

The most complex model takes the interaction of the valve leaflets with the blood flow into account [1, 17, 24, 50, 94]. As such, it is expected to be the most physiological one, even though the geometry of the leaflets is often simplified. One reason, highlighted for example by Vellguth (2017), is the challenge in constructing the geometries. The FSI model is the only model that can assess parameters like the valve closure time and the leaflets' stress and strain. Unfortunately, it results by far in the highest computational costs (compare Chapter 2.3).

prosthetic MV model

Since the available prosthetic heart valves all have characteristics and movements different from the physiological valve, Bakar (2015) separates the literature dealing with them into an independent category. Nonetheless, from the numerical point of view, the available approaches found can be sorted into the four previous categories [16, 22, 91].

For a more complete overview of the current state of research, the literature that serves as basis for the discussion of Bakar (2015) is extendedly listed in Appendix A.4. Summarising the results found in the literature to a global conclusion, two MV models seem superior over the others. Firstly, the planar MV model is easy to implement, flexible in shape and positioning and capable of reproducing the expected flow characteristics. Secondly, the FSI MV model is the closest to the physiological behaviour of the valve and provides additional information in terms of strains and stresses in the valve. However, it is significantly more challenging in geometry construction, computational time and numerical stability (compare Chapter 2.3.3). If the fluid flow is of major interest, the geometry-prescribed MV model can replicate the results of the FSI MV model at comparably lower computational costs, since only the fluid domain has to be solved and no coupling convergence has to be fulfilled.

Based on the preceding reflections, the planar MV model is chosen to be compared to the geometry-prescribed MV model throughout the following chapters.

6.2 Planar Geometry-Prescribed Mitral Valve Model

As concluded in the previous section, the planar MV model provides a large flexibility in terms of shape and positioning at low computational costs. As such, it is hypothetically suitable for an easy mimicking of the heart valves.

In this work, the approach is implemented into the idealised LV by means of a porous material law. Thereby, the blockage of porous medium cells that are inserted into the MV and aortic valve plane regulates the flow direction.

The area surrounded by the MV annulus is filled with a porous medium of which the porosity can be flexibly controlled. Thereby, the valve plane can be set to permeable, partly resistant or fully impermeable. If the whole valve plane is permeable or impermeable at once, this approach is equivalent to a diode type MV model. However, if the valve plane is split into multiple zones, as shown in Figure 6.1, a geometry prescription is enabled by means of a projection of the 3D valve onto the 2D plane.

For the cells included in the porous medium the describing equations have to be adjusted accordingly. A typical continuum approach for creeping flows ($\mathrm{Re} \ll 1$) is the linear Darcy law [111], where porosity effects are described in average over the porous volume

$$u_i = -\frac{k_p}{\mu}\frac{\Delta p}{\Delta x_i}. \tag{6.6}$$

Here, the volume-averaged fluid velocity, u_i, is connected to the pressure gradient over the porous volume, $\frac{\Delta p}{\Delta x_i}$, via the permeability, k_p. The permeability varies between one, in the case of no resistance, and zero, in the case of high resistance. Because the heart flow involves flows where $\mathrm{Re} \gg 1$, inertial effects have to be taken into account. Therefore, the Darcy model is extended by an inertial term representing the kinetic energy. The result is the Darcy-Forchheimer law [43]

$$\frac{\Delta p}{\Delta x_i} = -\frac{\mu}{k_p}u_i - \beta \rho u_i^2. \tag{6.7}$$

The Forchheimer coefficient, β, has to be determined experimentally. However, the approach of implementing porous regimes into the heart flow is not meant to mimic a certain material behaviour. It is used to simulate blockage.

Therefore, the Forchheimer coefficient is set to values as high as 10^{15} in the case of impermeability. A validation of the porous media implementation in the utilised OpenFOAM-1.6-ext solver is found in Appendix A.5.

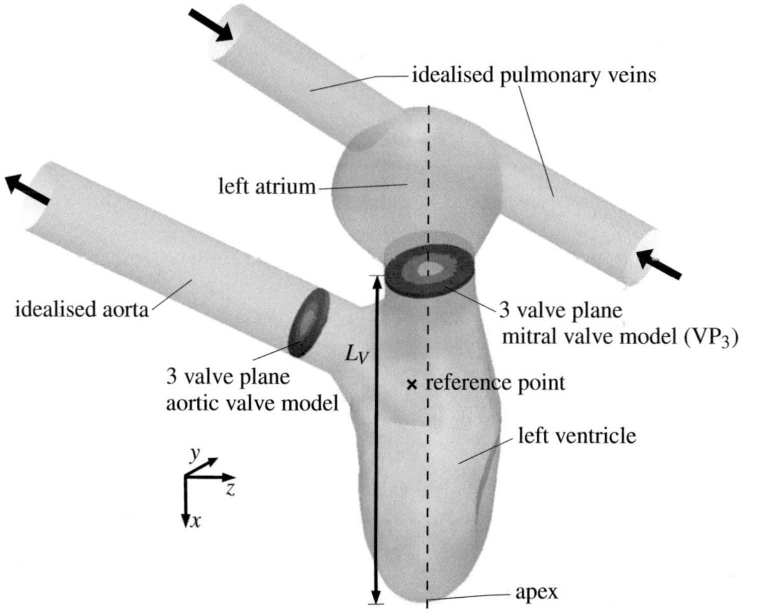

Figure 6.1: Simplified LV geometry at end systole with planar valve model. The dashed line marks the central axis connecting the atrium with the ventricle.

Figure 6.1 shows the simplified LV geometry with inserted porous cell regions in the MV and aortic valve plane. Positioning and orientation are chosen equal to respective physiological annulus positions [49]. In the simulations the outer porous ring stays closed at all times. As such, the effective opening area of a physiological valve is mimicked. This model configuration with three sections in the valve plane is abbreviated with VP_3. To illustrate the influence of the outer ring blockage, an additional test case is performed in the diode type configuration with only one porous zone in the valve plane, VP_1. First results of a comparison of the two configurations have been presented before

[SKF15]. They show good agreement with the results reported by Seo et al. [86], who highlight the necessity of inserting a more complex MV model than a simple diode type model.

One key question of this work deals with the validity of simplifications concerning the MV geometry model. As such, it is of interest to evaluate the sensitivity of the flow field characteristics on changes in the MV model. It is known that a deflection of the central axis between atrium an ventricle, indicated by the dashed line in Figure 6.1, significantly affects the vortex formation process [85]. A different influence has been presented [DKF16] where the central axis is not altered but the inclination of the MV plane itself. The presentation included three different tilting angles of the VP_3 MV model, which are measured with respect to the z-axis in Figure 6.1 as illustrated in Figure 6.2. The investigation covers the physiological original positioning, where the valve ring is tilted by $-6°$ towards the lateral wall, and two orientations that are oriented at an angle of $\alpha = 0°$ and $\alpha = 6°$. These tilting angles lie within the accuracy range that surgeons accomplish in MV replacement surgeries [31].

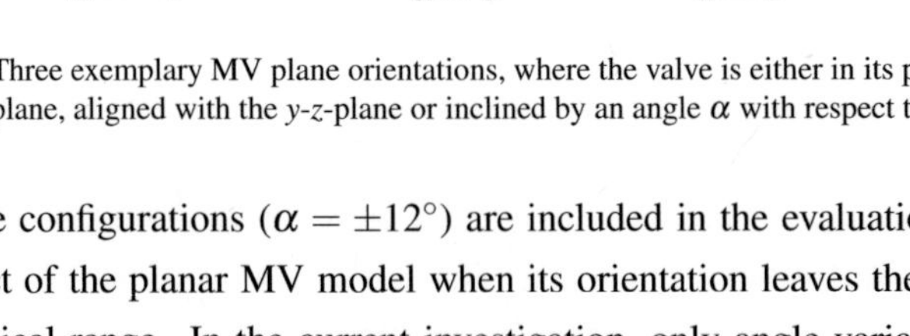

Figure 6.2: Three exemplary MV plane orientations, where the valve is either in its physiological plane, aligned with the y-z-plane or inclined by an angle α with respect to the z-axis.

Two more configurations ($\alpha = \pm 12°$) are included in the evaluations to test the impact of the planar MV model when its orientation leaves the expected physiological range. In the current investigation, only angle variations with respect to the z-axis are regarded. The choice of this approach is based on the positioning of the MV leaflets whose tips open and close parallel to the connecting line between aortic valve and lateral wall. It is hypothesised that changing the orientation of the VP_3 model along this axis (equal to the z-axis in the chosen coordinate system) can replicate the guiding influence of the MV leaflets onto the blood flow. The different configurations are distinguished by adding the angle to the specification, i.e. $VP_{3,\alpha}$.

As mentioned before, the pressure at the aorta and the pulmonary veins is prescribed. Two different approaches for pressure fixation are compared. On the one hand a constant value at all times and on the other hand a time varying value which is closer replicating the physiological system. The time-dependent evolution is determined with a model of the circulatory system developed by Reik et al. [75]. It receives the volume change of the ventricle as boundary condition and reproduces the arterial network of the circulatory systems with electrical analogies. Thereby, the implemented resistances yield the pressure values required for the heart flow computation. The resultant pressure boundaries are shown in Figure 6.3. The constant boundary value is chosen equal to the mean value of the time varying pressure.

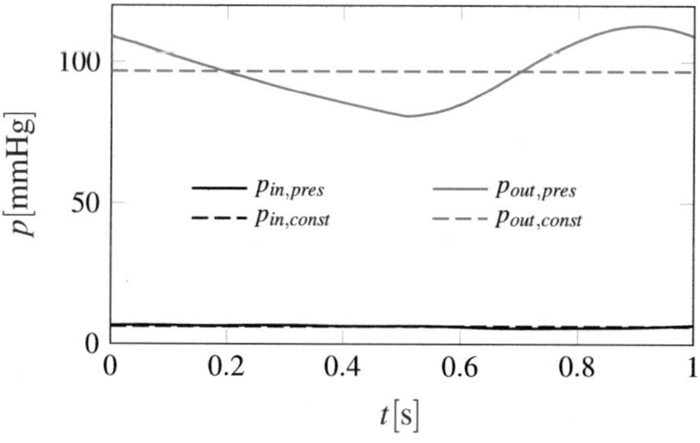

Figure 6.3: Two pressure boundary conditions that are applied in LV simulation. The pressure is either kept constant at inlet and outlet or varies with time.

As the LV wall movement is prescribed, the volume change of the geometry is equal in all configurations (see Figure 6.4). In contrast, the evolution of the mean pressure in the LV changes according to the boundary conditions. With the constant pressure boundary the pressure in the ventricle reaches its maximum at the end of the iso-volumetric contraction and then decreases nearly linearly during the whole systole. The prescribed pressure boundary results in a rising pressure over most of the systolic phase with its maximum during the late systole.

	W_{pV} **for** p_{bc} **constant**	W_{pV} **for** p_{bc} **prescribed**
$\mathbf{VP}_1$	$2120.7\,\mathrm{m^5\,s^{-2}}$	$2216.4\,\mathrm{m^5\,s^{-2}}$
$\mathbf{VP}_3$ and $\mathbf{VP}_{3,\alpha}$	$2259.8\,\mathrm{m^5\,s^{-2}}$	$2354.8\,\mathrm{m^5\,s^{-2}}$

Table 6.1: Pressure-volume work executed by the LV in dependency of the valve plane configuration and the pressure boundary condition. The pressure is scaled by the density $\rho = 1055\,\mathrm{kg\,m^{-3}}$.

Determining the pressure-volume work, W_{pV}, yields a lower value in the constant configuration compared to the prescribed pressure configuration. This is shown when comparing the areas within the pressure-volume curves in Figure 6.4. Because the diode type model introduces less blockage into the valve planes, the ventricle has to provide less pressure-volume work. Further, W_{pV} rises if the pressure boundary changes with time although the mean values at the boundaries are equal. This results from the fact that the ventricle has to overcome the resistance executed by the high pressure in the aorta during the systole which is significantly higher in the pressure prescribed configuration. Absolute values for the pressure-volume work are listed in Table 6.1. All values are determined using the calculated LV pressure which is scaled by the blood density, $\rho = 1055\,\mathrm{kg\,m^{-3}}$. This scaling is part of the OpenFOAM framework for incompressible solvers.

Only the results obtained with the pressure prescribed boundary are presented in the following evaluations, because the two boundary conditions do not yield significant differences in terms of vortex formation and progression.

For basic understanding of the flow vortices, the Q-criterion is analysed. It has to be kept in mind that it does not reveal clear vortex boundaries as the choice of the iso-value for visualisation is quite arbitrary. In the case of the VP_1 configuration, the Q-criterion does not detect clearly visible areas of rotation and hence no vortices. As such, it proves that the diode type MV model is not suitable for generating physiological flow conditions.

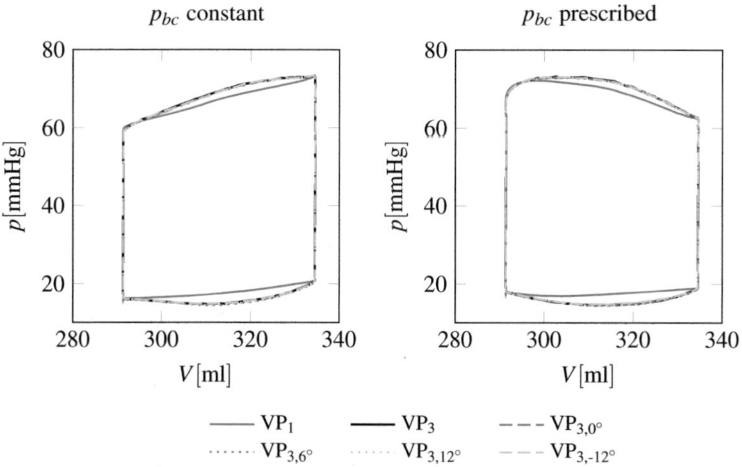

Figure 6.4: Pressure-volume diagrams for two different pressure boundary conditions and various MV plane orientations. The volume includes the volume of the atrium and the inlet and outlet branches.

Figure 6.5 shows iso-surfaces of the Q-criterion for VP_3, $VP_{3,-12°}$ and $VP_{3,12°}$ that represent the physiological and the two extreme cases. Vortices for $\alpha = 0°$ and $\alpha = 6°$ are located between the visualised cases and do not reveal additional information. At mid diastole ($t = 4.25\,s$), the vortex wake that is generated in the systolic phase of the previous heart beat is still present in front of the aortic valve. This wake is less dominant for tilting angles $\alpha > 0°$. When the ventricle starts expanding in the early diastolic phase, a vortex ring is detected behind the MV plane for all orientations. The formation is triggered by the vorticity in the inner and outer boundary layer of the outer porous cell zone. The ejection of the fluid jet from the atrium into the LV causes rising velocity gradients between the accelerated blood jet and the nearly resting blood in the chamber. Thereby, a vorticity flux is generated which feeds the growing vortex ring until it detaches from the valve ring. At the same time, the vortex wake in front of the aortic valve pushes the vortex ring towards the lateral wall.

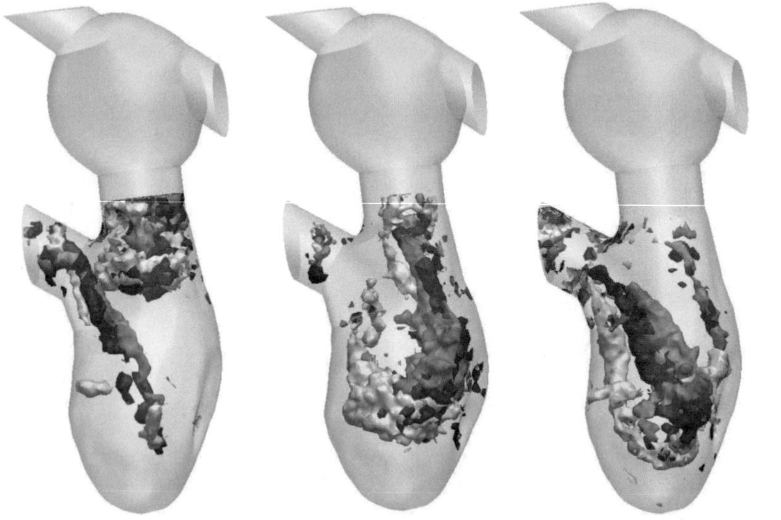

Figure 6.5: Time evolution of iso-surfaces at $Q = 300$ for the physiological and the two MV plane orientations with the largest tilting angles.

The typical tilting of the vortex can be seen at $t = 4.5\,\mathrm{s}$ for $\alpha \leq 0^\circ$. It is generated by the influence of the lateral wall which exerts friction and thus takes up some of the kinetic energy of the jet. For $\alpha > 0^\circ$ the vortex is stretched around its central axis, as the kinetic energy of the incoming fluid is less pronounced to friction and has to proceed somewhere when it approaches the apex. Afterwards, the ventricle starts contracting and guides the blood in a helical motion into the aorta which is detected by the Q-criterion in form of the typical vortex wake. This vortex wake at the end of the systole is present in all configurations, but its rotational flow component gets weaker with a growing tilting angle.

Overall, all VP_3 cases show the expected heart flow characteristics with differences in position and size. How much the velocity profile and thus the kinetic energy is shifted by different valve plane orientations is clarified by extraction of chosen velocity profiles. Figure 6.6 shows the time evolution of the velocity component in x-direction over a line positioned centrally below the MV plane and oriented parallel to the z-axis. At this position the x-component of the velocity is the main contributor to the kinetic energy. It can be seen that the incoming jet is shifted from being centred in the valve plane at $\alpha = 0°$ towards an asymmetric shape. The exact shape is dependent on the magnitude and direction of the inclination. An increasing angle generates increasing asymmetry whereby the kinetic energy is shifted towards the lateral wall when $\alpha > 0°$ and towards the interventricular septum when $\alpha < 0°$ (compare Figure 6.6). The findings leave the question unanswered how the energy shift in the MV plane influences the jet propagation in the LV.

The visualisation of the Q-criterion suggests that the whole jet direction is shifted according to the shift in the MV plane. In the original orientation ($\alpha = -6°$), the jet travels parallel to the lateral wall. In the case of $\alpha \geq 0°$ it is developing towards the ventricular apex. This is confirmed by contouring the x-velocity profile along the central axis between atrium and ventricle (compare dashed line in Figure 6.1). Figure 6.7 shows the time evolution of the corresponding velocity profile in x-direction. In all cases, the maximum velocity, $u_{max} = 0.8\,\mathrm{m\,s^{-1}}$, is reached at 4.25 s when the ventricular wall movement reaches the highest acceleration in the mid diastole. The velocity peak is located in close proximity to the blockage of the MV ring. For $\alpha = 6°$, the jet follows the central axis nearly linearly with time.

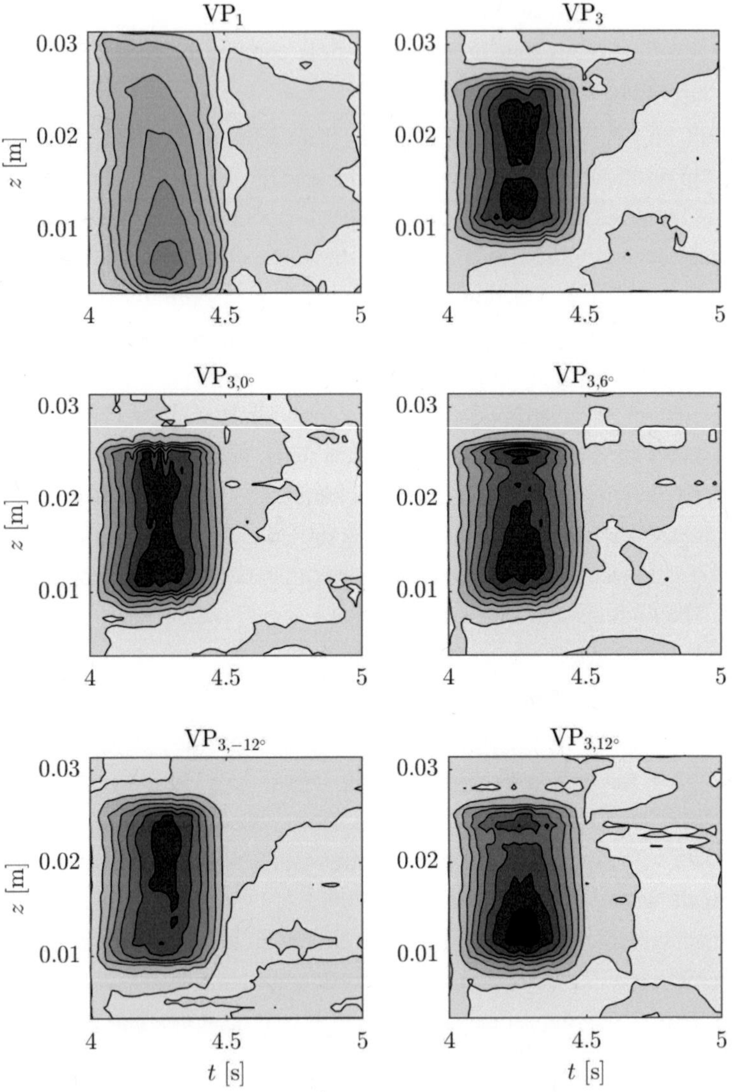

Figure 6.6: Time evolution of x-velocity behind the MV plane for different valve plane configurations, with velocities between $u_{min} = -0.1\,\mathrm{m\,s^{-1}}$ (white) to $u_{max} = 0.8\,\mathrm{m\,s^{-1}}$ (black).

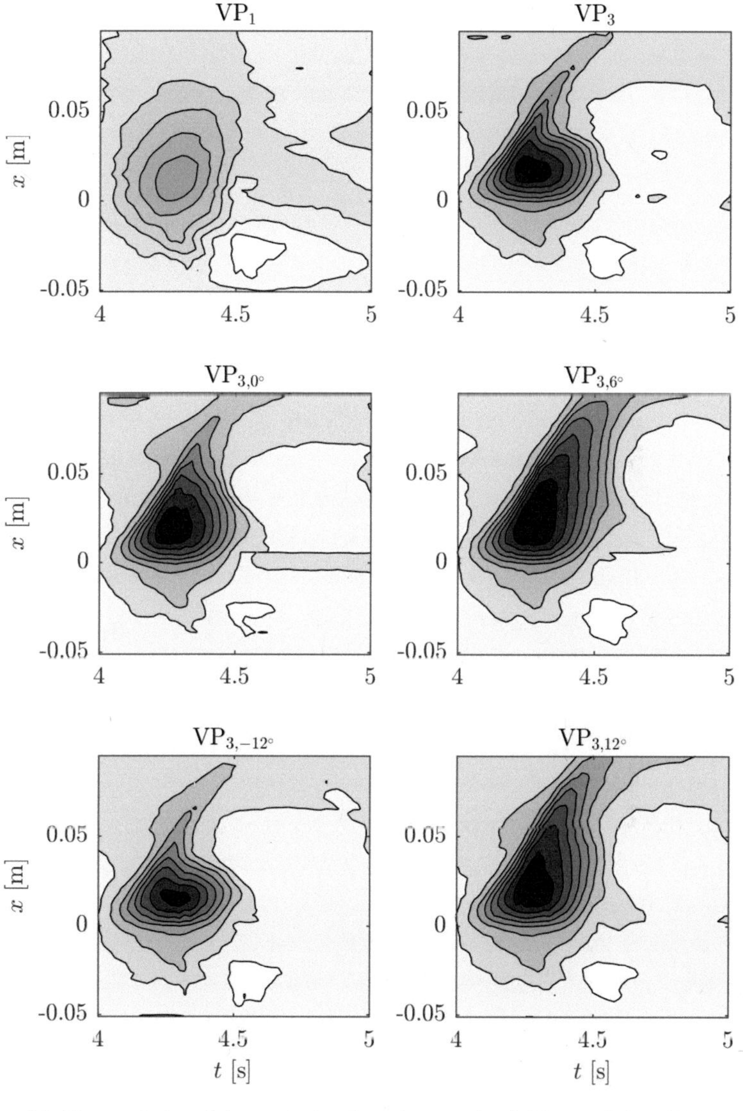

Figure 6.7: Time evolution of the x-velocity along the central axis between LA and LV for different valve plane configurations, with velocities reaching from $u_{min} = -0.1\,\mathrm{m\,s^{-1}}$ (white) to $u_{max} = 0.8\,\mathrm{m\,s^{-1}}$ (black).

With decreasing tilting angle, the presence of high velocity on the central axes decreases as the jet leans towards the lateral wall. This effect is less pronounced for $\alpha = 12°$. Although the amount of high velocity is reduced in comparison to $\alpha = 6°$, the amount of reduction is less compared to the other tilting angles.

These observations leave the answer to the question open, whether a proper washout of the ventricle takes place. The determination of LCS enables the detection of recirculation zones that would indicate an incomplete washout. Applying the resolution testing tools for the FTLE method developed in Chapter 5, namely the sum criterion and the relative error criterion, results in $PP = 23$, $VP = 23$ and $TP = 100$ in terms of sufficient particle and spatial and temporal data resolution (Brakhage (2016)). In accordance with the determined dimensionless numbers, the diameter of the MV, d_{MV}, is chosen as characteristic length scale. As such, those values are chosen for the post-processing. The slope evolutions of the testing criteria are similar compared to the results obtained for the double gyre flow and the von Kàrmàn vortex street. Thereby, the applicability of the criteria is further consolidated. Because of the flow periodicity, the integration time is chosen to be equal to the length of one period, $T_{int} = 1\,\mathrm{s}$.

Extracting LCS from backward FTLE fields enables the visualisation of blood volume that enters the heart. If the particles are tracked for a second heart beat, also the blood volume that entered during the previous heart beat can be extracted. The resultant 3D LCS are shown in Figure 6.8 for $\mathrm{VP_1}$ and $\mathrm{VP_3}$ at three different time points. At mid diastole, the jet of the $\mathrm{VP_3}$ configuration is already propagated deeper into the LV compared to $\mathrm{VP_1}$. Because the Q-criterion does not detect dominating rotation (compare Figure 6.5), the LCS that covers the current inflow of $\mathrm{VP_1}$ is mainly resultant from the shear stresses at the geometry walls. Following the current inflow LCS, the propagation of the vortex ring is clearly visible at the end diastole ($t = 4.5\,\mathrm{s}$) for $\mathrm{VP_3}$. At $t = 4.75\,\mathrm{s}$ the current inflow volume is passing along the apex and only small portion of the fresh blood is directly leaving the ventricle during the current heart beat. This indicates a proper washout and a smooth transition between diastole and systole. In contrast, the blood volume entering the heart in the VP_1 case does not pass along the apex and a significant portion is immediately leaving the LV. Also, no blood volume that entered during the previous cycle is detected close to the apex. This leads to the conclusion that old blood is recirculating in that zone. Tracking particles during four heart beats reveals that 46% of the blood in the LV is older than four cycles (see Table 6.2).

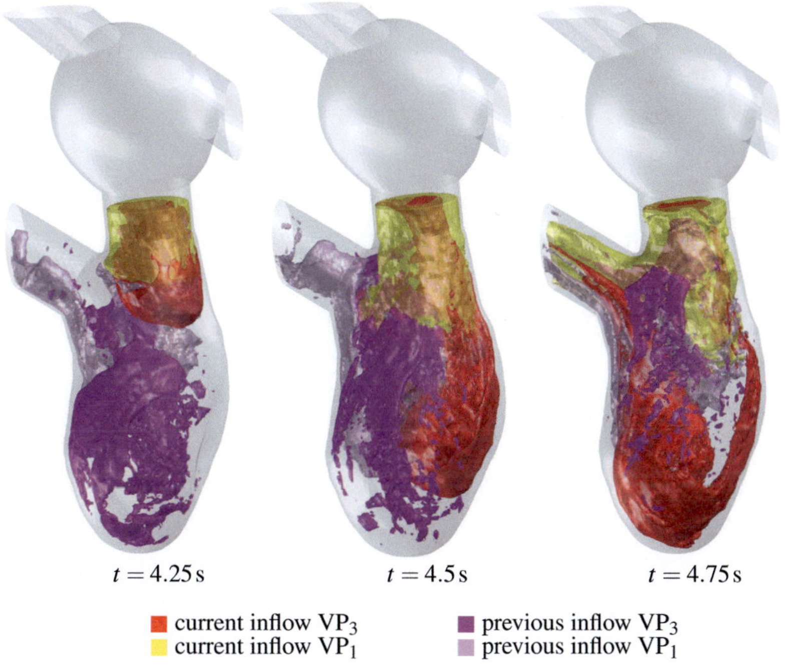

Figure 6.8: Extracted backward LCS wrapping the blood volume that enters the heart during the current beat or entered during the previous beat. Colour coding symbols either the VP_3 or the VP_1 model.

These findings are confirmed by extracting forward LCS (see Figure 6.9). They separate the blood volume that leaves the current heart beat from the volume that stays inside. Tracking the particles for a second heart beat highlights the fluid that leaves the heart in the following beat. In the VP_1 model the marked volume regions do not cover areas close to the apex but reach up into the atrium. Instead of guiding older blood from previous cycles into the circulatory system, the pumping process directly redirects a significant portion of fresh blood from the atrium into the aorta such that no mixing is enhanced and long particle residence times are expected.

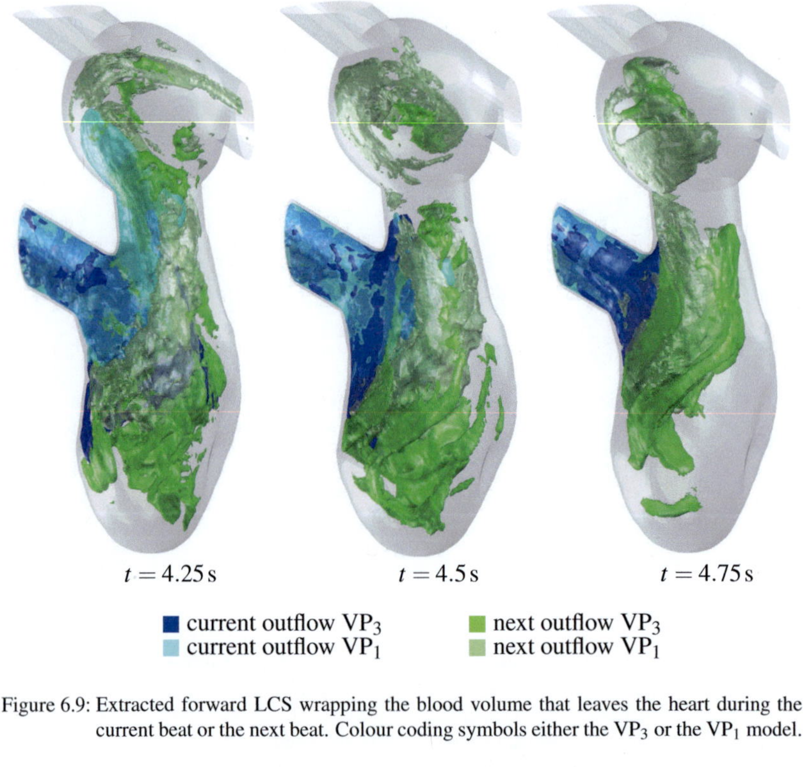

Figure 6.9: Extracted forward LCS wrapping the blood volume that leaves the heart during the current beat or the next beat. Colour coding symbols either the VP_3 or the VP_1 model.

Determining the volume that is included in a forward and a backward LCS reveals that 35% of the entering blood leaves the heart during the same beat. In case of VP_3 this share is about 9%. Here, the volume leaving the heart in two consecutive cycles is spread around the whole ventricle, which shows mixing of the entering blood and washout of the apex (compare Figure 6.9).

For comparison of the VP_3 model at different tilting angles, slices through the resulting LCS are compared at three different times in Figure 6.10. It can be seen that the jet changes its direction depending on the tilting angle, but overall the structures appear to be similar. These findings are in accordance with the results of the Q-criterion. Until the mid diastole, all VP_3 configurations show the same LCS development that marks the entering blood volume and the border of the developing vortex ring behind the blockage in the MV plane. In the midpoint of the cycle, the LCS lean towards the lateral wall and the vortex boundary close to the apex marks the rotation and stretching of the vortex. With increasing MV plane angle, α, the stretching of the LCS reaches in direction of the ventricular septum. Nonetheless, all depicted LCS arrive at the apex during the systolic phase, such that the blood from previous cycles is washed out smoothly.

From these observations the following question arises: How important are the differences in flow characteristics within the LCS for the circulatory system and especially on the risk of blood clotting and thrombus formation? The particle residence time that can give answers to this question is determined via the forward LCS extraction. The identified volumes within the LCS mark the volumes leaving the heart in consecutive heart beats. Table 6.2 lists the volume portions of the ventricular volume at the end of the diastole that leave the LV during four heart beats. The volume that is afterwards left in the heart consists of particles with residence times larger than four cycles. The flow field information needed for the particle tracking over four heart beats is solely taken from the last simulated heart beat which represents a periodic flow condition. Thus, the four tracking cycles have the same underlying velocity.

As already discussed, the particle residence times in VP_1 are significantly higher compared to VP_3. Further, it has to be noted that the particle tracking during the FTLE calculation tends to loose particles during the systolic phase if the ventricular wall passes over a particle located in close proximity to the boundary. These are the reasons why the volumes exerted during the first beat in Table 6.2 are not consistent and not equal to 23 %, which is the expected ejection fraction and should hold during the first beat. Nonetheless, a clear trend can be detected. The amount of leaving particles decreases from beat to beat as the pumping process mixes the older volume with the freshly entering blood. From the particles present in the ventricle at the start of the tracking, approximately 35% are left after the fourth beat for all VP_3 configurations. Without discussing every number in detail, it is seen that the numbers are very similar for the different valve orientations. As such, the variation of the valve orientation is not influencing the particle residence time.

The results show that significant differences in the flow patterns, e.g. comparing VP_1 and VP_3, have a measurable impact on the mixing of the freshly oxygenated atrial blood and the blood that resides in the ventricle at the beginning of any cycle. The generated washout correlates with reduced blood cell residence time in the ventricle. The washout is enhanced in the presence of a blockage in the MV annulus and it is robust to changes in valve plane orientation.

	1st beat	**2nd beat**	**3rd beat**	**4th beat**	**left volume**
$\mathbf{VP_1}$	20.9 %	15.52 %	9.99 %	7.59 %	46 %
$\mathbf{VP_3}$	21.35 %	20.41 %	14.6 %	9.28 %	34.36 %
$\mathbf{VP_{3,0^\circ}}$	21.42 %	19.82 %	14.71 %	10 %	34.05 %
$\mathbf{VP_{3,6^\circ}}$	21.77 %	20.18 %	14.06 %	8.91 %	35.08 %
$\mathbf{VP_{3,12^\circ}}$	21.63 %	19.71 %	14.87 %	9.53 %	34.26 %
$\mathbf{VP_{3,-12^\circ}}$	22.19 %	18.66 %	13.73 %	9.28 %	36.13 %

Table 6.2: Volume exerted in consecutive heart beats under variation of the planar MV model.

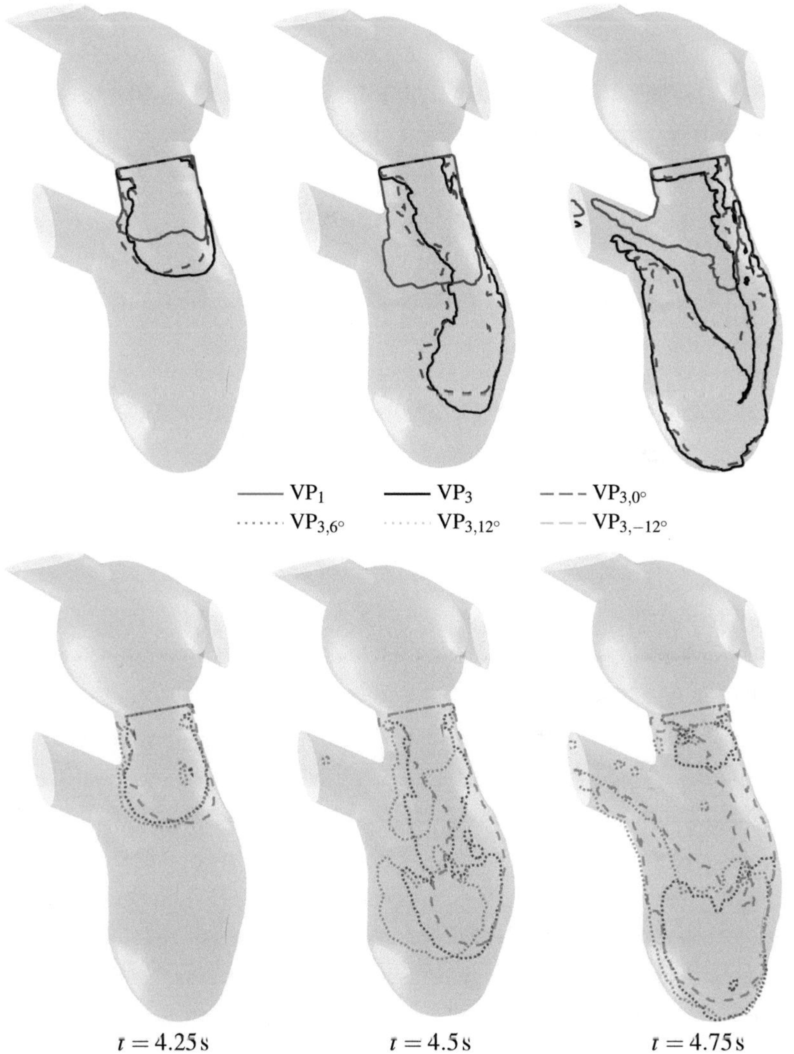

Figure 6.10: Slices through the resulting extracted LCS. The cut is positioned in the x-z-plane.

In a healthy human, a blood particle stays in the heart for no more than six cycles. Thus, the results obtained here seem very poor. However, a healthy EF of $60-70\%$ [92] pumps about three times more blood into the circulatory system in one beat compared to the current setting. With respect to the poor EF the results of the obtained particle residence time are realistic and prove the working conception of the planar MV model.

6.3 Geometry-Prescribed Mitral Valve Model

Although the planar MV model is capable of reproducing physiological flow characteristics and reasonable particle residence times, several research groups highlight the necessity of implementing 3D leaflets in the LV [8, 50, 60, 86, 103]. However, a 3D valve geometry has to be constructed and its movement has to be determined a priori or through computationally challenging FSI simulations. In this work, the simpler method is chosen, namely the prescribed motion that still requires more preparation and computational time compared to the planar MV model. Therefore, the behaviour of the VP_3 model is to be compared to a geometry-prescribed (geom.-pres.) approach.

The generated 3D valve is based on the simplified MV constructed by Seo et al. [86] and can be seen in Figure 6.11. The 2D basis shape on the left is rolled into a cylindrical shape and then bent towards its centre line. The resultant valve has an end diastolic height of 1.8 cm with a posterior leaflet length of 2 cm. At the end diastole (compare Figure 6.11) the angle between the posterior leaflet and the MV annulus plane measures $70.2°$. The whole valve is assumed to have a uniform thickness of 1.2 mm, which is slightly thicker than the normal range of 1 mm [37]. It is chosen to be larger than the fluid mesh resolution such that the immersed valve thickness cuts two fluid cells. Otherwise, one IB cell incorporates two boundaries which would require special treatment.

Since the valve is constructed in its open position, the closed state is yet to be found. Therefore, a mechanical simulation is conducted, in which the outer surface of the leaflets is loaded with a traction boundary condition. Figure 6.12 a) shows the applied absolute traction distribution in y- and z-direction that increases with darkening grey-scale. The maximum traction prescribed reaches $5350\,\mathrm{kg\,m^{-1}\,s^{-2}}$, which agrees very well with physiological forces acting on the heart valves [4]. Within this framework, the traction boundary condition represents a Neumann boundary condition for the solid movement, as it contributes to the displacement gradient [98]. While the leaflets are pushed towards each other to force the valve to close, the commissures are set under a tension which stunts them from collapsing. Thereby, a turn-down of the valve into the atrium is suppressed and thus the task of the neglected papillary muscles and chordae tendineaes is replaced.

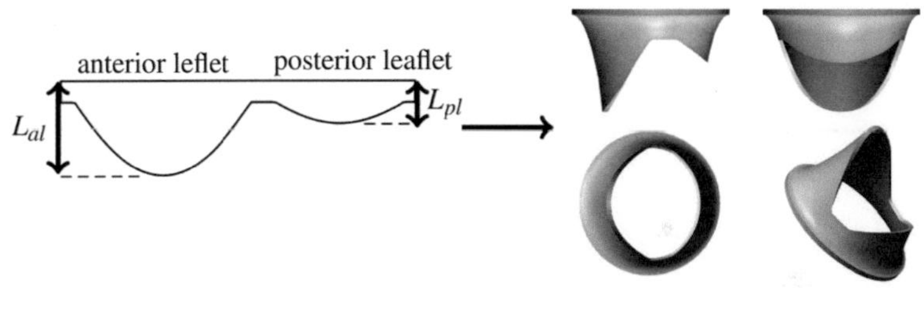

Figure 6.11: Generated 3D MV for the geom.-pres. MV model. The geometry is based on the descriptions in [86].

The annulus ring is rigid and forced to stay in place at all times. This simplification is only valid in the case of a steady atrium. The simulation is conducted using the solid mechanics framework included in foam-extend 3.1 that applies the finite volume method. An extension by Gollub (2013) enables the usage of a non-linear total Lagrangian approach that realises an isotropic hyper-elastic Saint Venant-Kirchhoff material. Following the guideline of De Hart et al. [18], the density of the structural material, ρ_s, is set equal to the blood density ($\rho_s = \rho = 1055\,\mathrm{kg\,m^{-3}}$) and the Young's modulus is set to $E = 1.5 \cdot 10^6\mathrm{kg\,m^{-1}\,s^{-2}}$. In order to increase the numerical stability, which is fragile due to the large movement, bending and folding of the structure, the Poisson ratio is reduced from the physiological value of 0.49 to $\nu_s = 0.3$. The determined closed valve is shown in Figure 6.12 b).

The resulting closure phase length of 0.25 s matches the half length of the diastolic phase. Since no contact model is included in the simulation, the two leaflet tips overlap at full closure (compare Figure 6.12 b)). 25 geometries are stored and used for prescribing the closure and – backwards – the opening of the valve in the IBM simulations. Necessary information at time steps between the stored steps is determined through cubic spline interpolation.

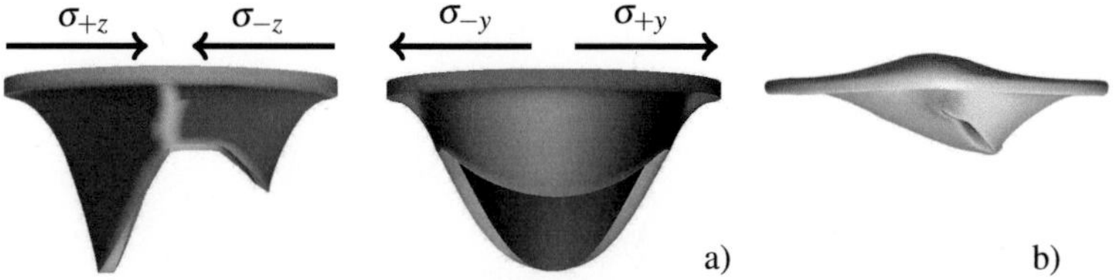

Figure 6.12: a) Traction boundary condition for the solid mechanics simulation of the 3D MV movement with $|\sigma_{\pm y}|_{max} = 5350\,\mathrm{kg\,m^{-1}\,s^{-2}}$ (darkest shadowing, light grey symbols traction free). b) MV at its closed state after $t = 0.25\,\mathrm{s}$.

The 3D MV is inserted into the already introduced idealised LV such that the anterior leaflet is positioned next to the aorta wall and the posterior leaflet is positioned next to the lateral wall. The simulation is conducted in an IB framework where the mesh resolution is chosen such that 200,000 cells lie inside of the ventricle. The resulting resolution of the equidistant mesh is $\Delta x = \Delta y = \Delta z = 1\,\mathrm{mm}$ which yields a total of 1,316,250 cells. In the flow simulation, full closure of the MV is not realisable so far because of two reasons. Firstly, the overlapping of the leaflets causes instabilities in the continuity equation. Secondly, when an IB cell is next to both leaflets, e.g. close to the commissures between the leaflets, it receives contradictory information.

Since the valve closure cannot be used to guide the flow direction, the boundary conditions are adapted accordingly. Here, the inlet veins are blocked by a no-slip condition during the systolic phase and the aorta is blocked during the diastole. Without the internal resistance of the porous media model, the physiological pressure difference between atrium and aorta cannot be maintained. Thus, only a pressure rise from the pulmonary veins to the aorta of $\frac{\Delta p}{\rho} = 1\,\mathrm{m}^2\,\mathrm{s}^{-2} \widehat{=} 7.91\,\mathrm{mmHg}$, with $\rho = 1055\,\mathrm{kg}\,\mathrm{m}^{-3}$, is realised. It is about ten times lower compared to normal conditions. Three consecutive heart beats are simulated to save computational time. This approach is considered valid for the present evaluation, since the changes observed in the flow characteristics between the last two consecutive heart beats are significantly smaller compared to the differences between the 3D MV and the planar MV model. Consequently, the third simulated cycle is used for the following analyses.

Figure 6.13 shows the resulting Q-criterion with positive (red) and negative (blue) iso-surfaces. The vortex ring formation is clearly visible at mid diastole. Further, a region of dominating strain is located in close proximity of the vortex ring, where the high velocity jet is in friction with the nearly resting fluid in the LV. A tilting motion of the vortex is observed at mid diastole and remains present until the end of this phase. At this stage, dominating strain regions are detected along the whole lateral wall. During the systole, the fluid leaves the ventricle in its typical helical movement, shown by the red smooth elongated iso-surface. Another vortex is detected close to the 3D valve. It is generated at the anterior leaflet during valve closure and is kept in motion by the helical structure close by during the systolic phase. The few spots of dominating strain lead to the conclusion that a smooth ejection takes place.

Due to the same framework and the similar available velocity resolution, the parameters for LCS extraction are equal to the settings in the previous section. The resultant backward and forward LCS are shown for two consecutive heart beats in Figure 6.14. During the diastole, the anterior MV leaflet guides the incoming jet towards the lateral wall. At the leaflet tip, a vortex starts rolling up that consists of freshly entering blood mixing with already present older blood. Further, at $t = 4.25\,\text{s}$, it can be seen that the blood volume which entered in the previous beat partially overlaps with the LCS that mark the outflow for two heart beats. Thus, the blood close to the apex is washed out within three cycles. A proper washout of the ventricle is confirmed when the current inflow is further regarded at the end diastole. Here, the entering jet reaches the apex of the LV. During the systolic phase, the connectivity of the entering blood volume is further breaking down, which signals a good mixing behaviour of the flow.

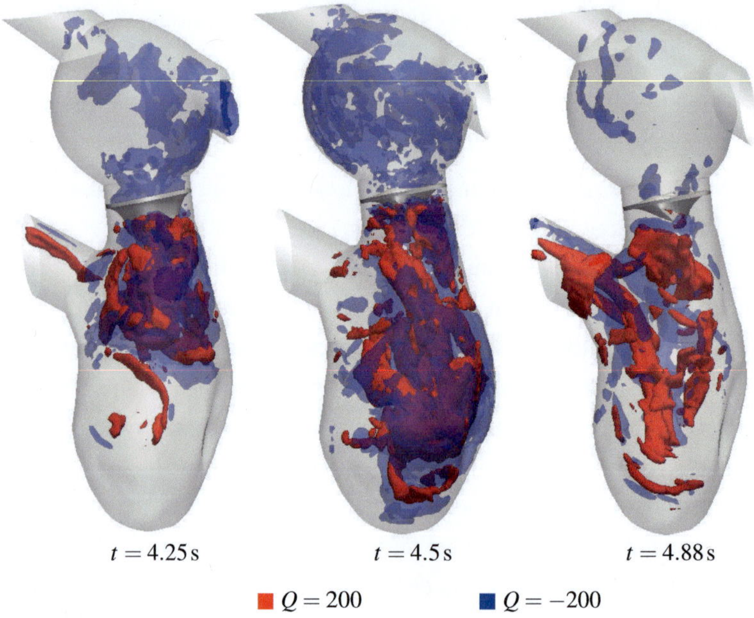

Figure 6.13: Time evolution of iso-surfaces at (red) $Q = 200$ marking regions of dominating rotation and (blue) $Q = -200$ marking regions of dominating strain with the geom.-pres. MV model.

In comparison to the VP_3 model, the detected structures in terms of Q-criterion and LCS extraction appear to have less sharp borders signalling a more chaotic flow with supposedly enhanced mixing. Reliable conclusions on particle residence times and thus pumping efficiency have to be based on FTLE analyses that incorporate at least four heart beats such that the total amount of ejected blood volume equals the ventricular volume. Then, the portion of old blood left in the heart gives insight into potential particle residence times. Therefore, the last simulated cycle, which is assumed to represent a periodic flow state, is used repeatedly for four cycles as basis for a particle tracking over four heart beats.

The usage of all simulated heart cycles would include the non-periodic, unphysiological starting flow field and thereby introduce avoidable errors. The results are presented in the next section and directly compared to the VP_3 model.

The structural flow differences between VP_3 and the geom.-pres. MV result not solely from the dimensional differences. Also, the effective opening areas in VP_3 and in the geom.-pres. model are neither similar in shape nor in size. These differences are eliminated in the following section by adapting VP_3 accordingly.

6.4 Sensitivity of Flow Characteristics on Chosen Valve Model

Seo et al. [86] underline their recommendation of implementing a geom.-pres. valve by comparing the resultant flow field in a patient specific LV with a diode type MV. The resultant flow field with the diode type MV is in agreement with the results for VP_1 presented in Section 6.2. Since the VP_3 model shows superior behaviour, it is compared to the geom.-pres. MV throughout this section.

As concluded previously, the shape of the planar model is adapted to mimic the effective opening area of the 3D valve in terms of shape and size. Figure 6.15 shows the planar MV model generated through projection of the 3D valve onto a 2D plane. The projection is performed at three different time steps during the first half of the diastole, i.e. at $t = 4$ s, $t = 4.1$ s and $t = 4.25$ s.

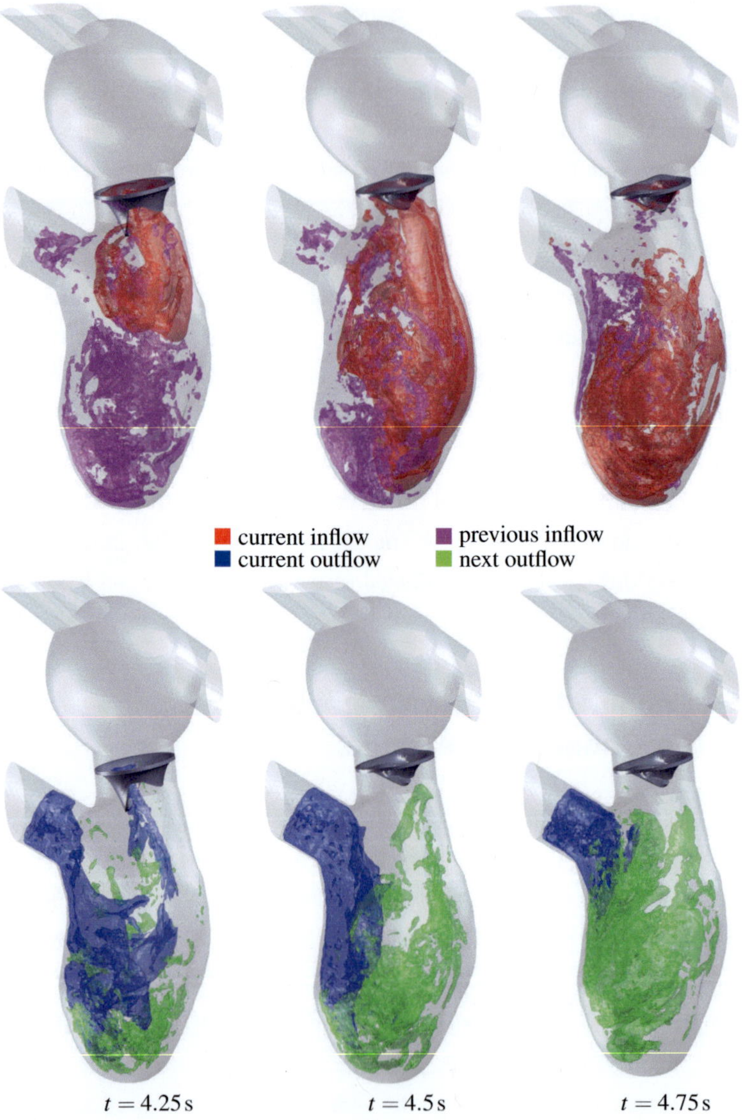

Figure 6.14: Extracted backward and forward LCS wrapping the blood volume that enters or leaves the ventricle with the geom.-pres. MV model.

Firstly, the valve is fully closed and a projection results in a fully blocked valve plane. Secondly, an early time point is chosen, where the opening area complies about half of the maximum opening area. Lastly, the widest opening at mid diastole is used for projection of the maximum effective opening area. The resultant projections are used to mark three different cell zones over the MV plane: the outer, the middle and the inner cell zone. The three zones are recognisable in Figure 6.15 (middle) as: dark grey that represents impermeable cells; light grey representing changing resistance; and white which highlights a permeable area. These three zones exist throughout the whole diastole. As soon as the ventricle starts relaxing at $t > 4\,\mathrm{s}$, the resistance of the inner cell zone is removed to let fluid pass through. Cells marked as resistant (light-grey) undergo a transition from impermeable to fully permeable during the valve opening ($4\,\mathrm{s} < t < 4.25\,\mathrm{s}$) and back to impermeable during valve closure phase ($4.25\,\mathrm{s} < t < 4.5\,\mathrm{s}$). As a first attempt, the transition is assumed to be linear. Other possibilities are conceivable, e.g. a dependency on exact valve movement, pressure differences over the MV plane or the volume flux.

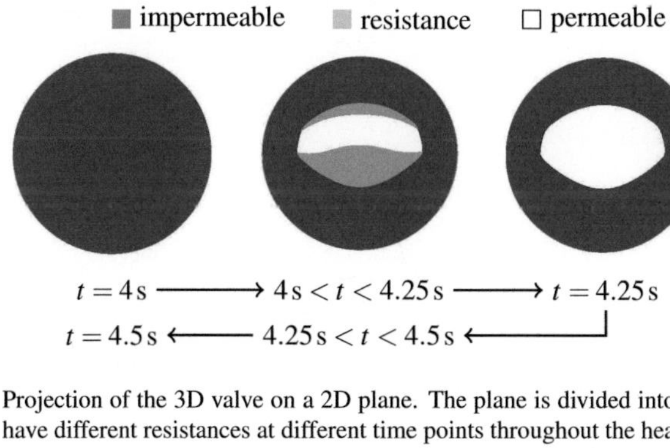

Figure 6.15: Projection of the 3D valve on a 2D plane. The plane is divided into three areas that have different resistances at different time points throughout the heart beat.

On the first glance, the iso-surfaces of $Q > 0$ and $Q < 0$ shown in Figure 6.16 seem to have no similarity to the corresponding results with the 3D valve. However, several things have to be kept in mind when interpreting the results. Firstly, the 3D valve simulation is carried out on a structured mesh and thus no interpolation of the velocity data is necessary for the post processing. In contrast, the unstructured velocity data of the planar valve model is interpolated linearly which induces minor errors into the flow field. Secondly, both the planar and the 3D MV are not a hundred percent equal to the physiological valve.

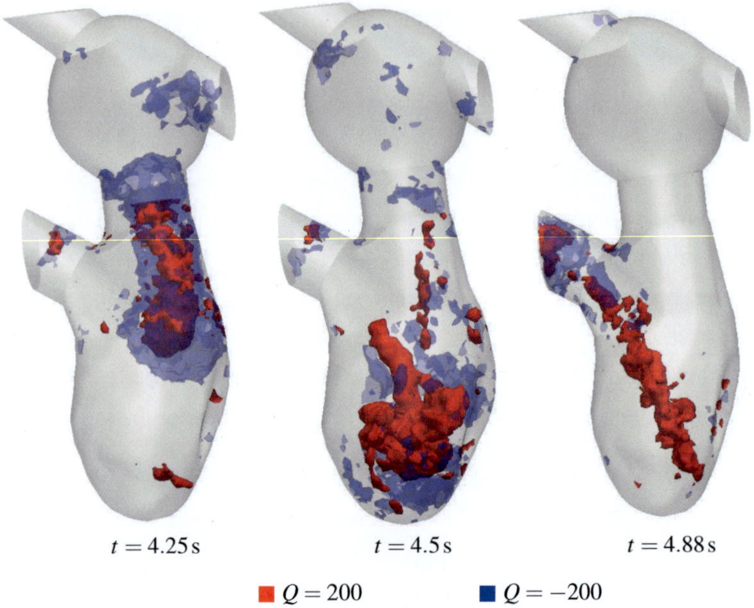

Figure 6.16: Time evolution of iso-surfaces at (red) $Q = 200$ marking regions of dominating rotation and (blue) $Q = -200$ marking regions of dominating strain with the planar MV model.

Although the generated vortex at the MV plane in Figure 6.16 is smaller compared to previous results, it follows the expected behaviour. At the early diastole it is guided towards the lateral wall, where it starts tilting and breaking. Simultaneously, a layer of dominating strain builds a hull around the vortex. Both iso-surfaces have travelled down into the apex at $t = 4.5\,\text{s}$, where they already lost in shape and connectivity. The strain zone seems to be more dissipative compared to the fluid rotation. In contrast, the 3D MV generates vortices and strain also in the upper half of the LV during the diastole. At $t = 4.88\,\mathrm{s}$ the typical helix is detected in the LV. However, no vortex is left close to the MV due to the missing leaflet.

Slices through the extracted LCS enable the direct comparison of the two LV models. Figure 6.17 shows detected backward LCS for three different time steps: mid-diastole, mid-heart beat and mid-systole. At mid-diastole, the differences in the initial jet building phase become clear. The planar model has a more narrow opening area, which increases the kinetic energy of the incoming jet. Therefore, the jet penetrates deeper into the ventricle. Further, the role-up of the fluid at the 3D leaflet tip is visible. This process cannot be reproduced to the same extent by the planar MV. However, both incoming LCS are guided towards the lateral wall, show the resultant tilting of the vortex-ring and reach into the apex at the end of the diastole ($t = 4.5\,\mathrm{s}$). During the systolic phase, the LCS show no similarities, at least in the slice regarded in Figure 6.17. Bearing in mind that a 2D slice only shows a small portion of the 3D information, the majority of the detected characteristics show similarities although they cannot be classified as equal.

Table 6.3 lists the volume portions that leave the ventricle during four consecutive heart beats for both MV models. In both cases, the last simulated periodic cycle serves as basis for the evaluation. Thus, the four tracking cycles have the same underlying velocity. The numbers underline the previous appearance of enhanced mixing with the 3D MV. In the first three beats, the leaving blood volumes are nearly similar, while the 3D valve shows superior behaviour in the fourth beat. Thus, the portion of old blood after the fourth beat is 3.67 % higher compared to the planar valve. Considering the high error that is currently present in the post-processing method, the results are not as different as they seem at first. As such, the comparison of the valve models reveals less optimisation in terms of washout performance than conveyed in the literature.

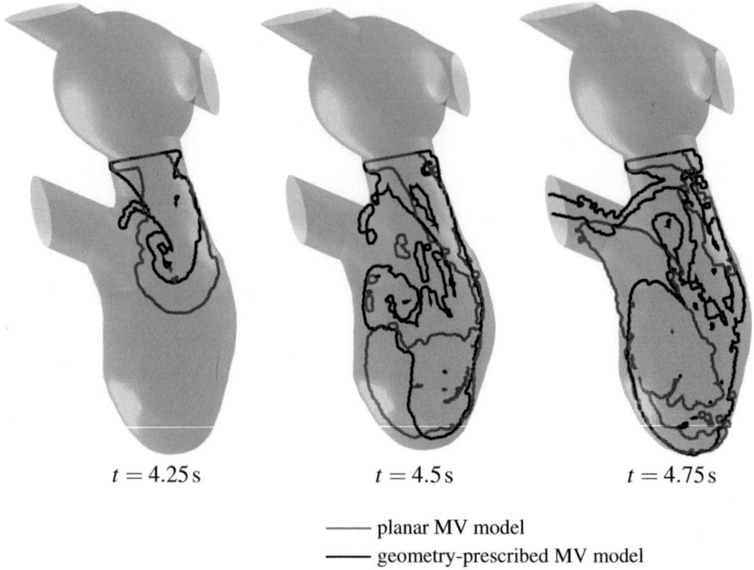

Figure 6.17: Slices through backward LCS extracted for two different MV models. The cut is positioned in the x-z-plane.

Concluding, the flow results for the planar model and geom.-pres. model evaluated with the Q-criterion and the FTLE differ from each other, but show similar flow characteristics and vortex formation. Both lead to physiological flow behaviour. However, evaluating the simulation costs, significant differences are found between the utilised solving procedures. Some statistics on the two different models are listed in Table 6.4.

	1st beat	**2nd beat**	**3rd beat**	**4th beat**	**left volume**
planar	21.64 %	17.44 %	13.21 %	9.41 %	38.3 %
geom.-pres.	20.22 %	18.35 %	13.85 %	12.95 %	34.63 %

Table 6.3: Volume exerted in consecutive heart beats incorporating the planar MV model and the geom.-pres. MV model.

Since wall movement is included in both cases, the same numerical solver settings are used (compare Appendix A.5). Both simulations are carried out with the PIMPLE algorithm that couples the solution of the momentum equation with the Poisson equation for the pressure correction over multiple cycles. The NSE are solved until the residuals drop below 10^{-6} and the pressure correction is solved until the residual drops below 10^{-5}. Due to the observed convergence rate, the IBM is set up to carry out four PIMPLE cycles, while the ALE only conducts two cycles. Additionally, one cycle in the IBM takes nearly 20 times longer compared to the ALE. The solution of the momentum equations in x-, y- and z-direction comprises about 15 % (IBM) and 30 % (ALE) of the PIMPLE calculation time. This difference results from the larger number of iterations necessary to derive the pressure correction in the IBM case. Further, the solution with the IBM is not optimised to solve the equations only in the fluid and the IB cells. The six times larger cell count leads to a six times longer computational time per single iteration and equation. As such, an optimisation by means of a flexible equation system size in dependency of the number of fluid cells has the potential to reduce the execution time of solving equations by a factor of 6. Since the PIMPLE loop additionally includes the correction of the boundary conditions, the time saving for the whole loop cannot reach this idealised factor to its full extend.

		execution times			
	cell count	one heart beat	solve momentum	PIMPLE loop	mesh -sort/ -motion
planar (ALE)	204,737	4.53 h	1.16 s	3.6 s	0.81 s
geom.-pres. (IBM)	1,316,250	116.19 h	10.34 s	70.35 s	17.97 s

Table 6.4: Statistics on the solvers for the planar MV model and the geom.-pres. MV model. Mean values are used for the execution times.

Both simulation techniques include tasks that are not necessary in the other. In the ALE (planar MV) the mesh motion has to be determined and in the IBM (geom.-pres. MV) the mesh cells have to be sorted into fluid, solid and IB cells. Solving the mesh motion shows fast convergence and is responsible for 9.93 % of the total computation time. The sorting algorithm in the IBM comprises 5.68 % of the total time needed (compare Table 6.4). It is responsible for detecting the IB cells and sorts all cells into the three categories, namely fluid, solid or IB cell. This procedure has to be repeated in each time step since the cells can change their affiliation in the moving boundary framework. However, the algorithm has the potential to be optimised to further reduce the computational time. Decreasing the time of the sorting algorithm has a growing impact on the total computational time-dependent on the optimisation of the PIMPLE loop. The current implementation loops over the full cell count in each time step. Instead, only the cells in close proximity of a moving boundary should be evaluated from the second time step on. 28,099 IB cells are identified in the presented heart geometry. Since the heart wall does not skip cells while moving, it is enough to evaluate the current IB cells and their direct neighbours. Dependent on the geometry of the IB surface, the number of cells for evaluation is about three times the number of IB cells. This reduces the sorting loop count to 6.4 % $\equiv$ 1.15 s after the initialisation.

With the first suggested optimisations, the computational time can be reduced remarkably. Nonetheless, another 5 % of the currently needed computational time in the IBM is used for the reading and writing processes of which the reading is negligibly small. Carefully taken decisions on which variables are stored and how often they are written sum up to the total writing time. In practical application, the storage of e.g. the IB marker fields is not necessary, while they can yield meaningful insights within the process of code development.

Summing up the suggested optimisations yields a possible decrease of the IBM calculation time of 80 %, which results in an execution time of approximately 21 h for one heart beat. As such, the ALE configuration with the planar

MV is still four times faster. It has to be kept in mind that these quantitative evaluations are based on statistics of a single core simulation on one specific platform and are not generally valid. Nonetheless, all conclusions are qualitatively meaningful.

Considering the rarely available necessary MRI resolution needed to generate an exact physiological MV, it is likely that the results with the idealised MV differ from the physiological valve in the same extend as they differ from the results with the planar model. That said, a time-dependent projection of the effective opening area from a patient specific geometry is easier to establish and can be implemented into an *in-silico* model in no time. Since the obtained flow characteristics match with the expected and the current computational effort is nearly 20 times lower, the planar MV model is implemented in a patient specific LV in the following chapter. Thereby, the applicability to a more complex scenario is proven.

7 Application to a Patient Specific Left Ventricle

This chapter presents an investigation of a more realistic patient-specific LV. It is meant to show the applicability of the planar MV model within a more physiological scenario and some numerical challenges that occur additionally to the ones mentioned so far. First, the model details and modelling challenges are summarised and then the simulation results are presented.

7.1 Model Description and Modelling Challenges

The geometry is generated from MRI data at the Institute of Biomedical Engineering of the Karlsruhe Institute of Technology using the procedure presented by Fritz et al. [26]. The data set includes one set of static 3D-information at diastole and multiple 2D-slices at various time steps throughout the heart cycle. Manual segmentation of the data enables the generation of a full heart model. It is used to simulate the muscular contraction as reaction to the electrical activation of the sinus node. The resultant ventricular movement is used for prescription of the wall movement that serves as boundary condition for the flow field simulation. Only the left side of a patient-specific heart is utilised here.

It comprises of the atrium and its four pulmonary veins and the LV. The extracted LV has an ejection fraction of $EF = \frac{V_{stroke}}{V_{dia}} = 47.7\,\%$, which is still lower than a healthy value of approximately $60-70\,\%$. Nonetheless, it is twice as much as in the idealised LV presented in Chapter 6 and therefore noticeably more realistic. One heart beat lasts 0.8 s whereof the diastole comprises the first 0.45 s. 160 surface geometries are available in the flow simulation for one heart beat. Since smaller time steps than 0.005 s have to be realised, the surface geometry needed at time steps in between the given ones is interpolated through cubic splines. The surface mesh is an a priori refinement of the original mesh used for the description of the structural deformation of the heart muscle at the Institute of Biomedical Engineering. Thereby, the boundary nodes are preserved such that not only the volume change is replicated but also the twisting motion of the ventricle is preserved.

The time-dependent pressures at the pulmonary veins and the aorta are assumed from the windkessel model in the structural simulations. Thus, they are prescribed in the fluid simulation at all time steps and the flux across the patches adjusts according to the volume change in the LV. Five consecutive heart beats are predicted with the fluid solver to generate a periodic flow.

In contrast to the previous model, the atrium and therefore also the MV plane are not fixed in space but move with time. Close to the end of the diastole, the atrium contracts and generates a second, weaker jet of blood entering into the ventricle. Due to the valve plane motion, the Darcy-Forchheimer porosity model in Equation (6.7) is not suitable anymore. It forces the flow to stagnate in the porous zone due to the high resistance but instead a model is needed that adds kinetic energy into the flow through its displacement. Hereby, the velocity within the porous zone is equal to its motion. The ALE framework is used, since the porosity zone is then automatically moving in dependency of the mesh motion and thus the valve plane displacement. A porosity model that fulfils the requirements has been developed by Wang et al. [107], where

$$F_p = -\frac{\nu \phi_p}{k_p}(u_i - c_i) - \frac{1.75\sqrt{\phi_p}}{\sqrt{150 k_p}}(u_i - c_i)\left|u_i - c_i\right|, \tag{7.1}$$

with $k_p = 10^{-13}\mathrm{m}^2$ being the permeability and $\phi_p = 1$ being the porosity. The resultant forcing term, F_p, is inserted into the NSE (2.5) and adjusts each time step in dependency of the mesh motion velocity, c_i, such that the velocity within the porous cell is forced to be equal to the mesh motion. Thereby, the moving porous zone in the MV plane functions like a moving wall with a no-slip boundary condition. The implementation of the model into the foam-extend 3.1 solver is validated in Appendix A.5. A direct insertion of a physical wall is numerically challenging, because the mesh would be cut into two independent meshes when the valve fully closes. As such, the topology of the mesh ought to be changed and boundary conditions for the pressure would have to be defined.

As guessed from Figure 7.1, the MV plane is not circular but has an ellipsoidal shape. Unfortunately, no information on the MV shape or the effective opening area is available. As such, the generation of an idealised 3D-MV with unknown shape and motion algorithm is not worth the effort. In contrast, adjusting the VP_3 model to form an ellipsoid is fast and easy. The blockage from the outer ring is chosen to be 25 %, such that the resultant maximum velocity reaches the physiological range with $u_{max} = 0.85\,\mathrm{m\,s^{-1}}$ and the time stepping during the simulation is manageable.

Further numerical challenges concern the mesh motion in the ALE configuration. Due to the higher ejection fraction and the moving valve plane, the boundary nodes and therefore also the inner cells have to undergo a considerably larger deformation compared to the previous case. Since numerical errors in the mesh motion lead to increasing non-orthogonality, cell openness and invalid cell volumes, the error should be kept small. A quadratic diffusivity to solve the mesh motion with Equation (2.11) has shown the best results in terms of mesh quality. In the current setup a time step of $\Delta t = 0.0002\,\mathrm{s}$ is necessary to maintain a good quality mesh and $CFL < 1$. Thereby, the simulation time for one heart beat of the patient specific ventricle results in 7.3 h, although the mesh comprises with 188,723 cells even less cells compared to the idealised LV used for the VP_3 model.

7.2 Resultant Flow Characteristics

Figures 7.1 and 7.2 show the flow results of the patient-specific LV geometry with the VP_3 MV model. The Q-criterion in Figure 7.1 highlights the generated ring vortex behind the MV plane during the diastole. It also shows that the vortex detaches and travels into the LV.

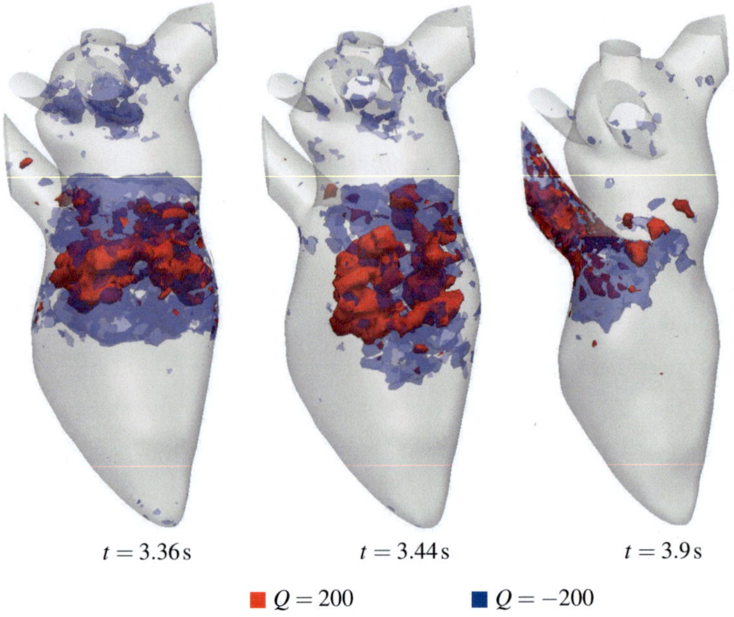

Figure 7.1: Time evolution of iso-surfaces at (red) $Q = 200$ marking regions of dominating rotation and (blue) $Q = -200$ marking regions of dominating strain with the planar MV model in a patient-specific LV.

Unlike in the idealised LV, the rotation of the fluid is not maintained until the inflowing jet reaches the apex. Instead, the vortex starts tilting early and fully breaks down. The apex seems to be too sharp to support a smooth filling to ejection transition. This observation is supported by the visualisation of the late systole, where the typical helical outflow is missing.

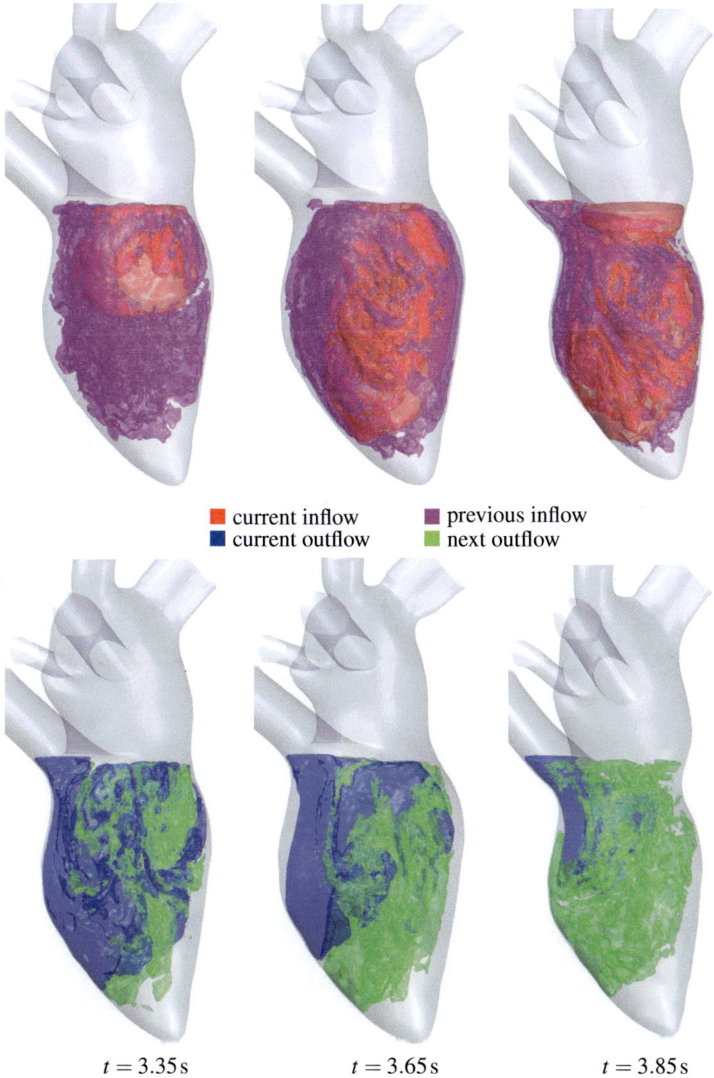

Figure 7.2: Extracted backward and forward LCS wrapping the blood volume that enters or leaves the ventricle for the patient specific ventricle with the planar MV model.

The question whether the washout is incomplete cannot be answered with the Q-criterion, as it does not uncover cause-effect relations or particle movement. Regions of dominating strain are found in the valve planes and at the tip of the jet as in the case of the idealised LV.

The extraction of LCS confirms that the incoming jet does not penetrate the whole apex (compare Figure 7.2). A small portion of the sharp tip does neither contain fresh blood from the last two cycles nor does it leave during the following cycles. The shape of the ventricle encourages a centred propagation of the incoming blood jet. Previously present fluid is pushed towards all sides of the ventricle and is not as smoothly guided towards the aorta as in the idealised LV. Nonetheless, a large volume close to the lateral wall and in the lower half of the ventricle is covered by forward and backward LCS, showing that the volume leaving during the current heart beat predominantly consists of blood from the previous cycle. No LCS is detected in the apex, which confirms the concerns fomented by the inspection of the Q-criterion, namely the missing washout of the apex.

	1st beat	**2nd beat**	**3rd beat**	**4th beat**	**left volume**
geom.-pres.	41.62 %	26.97 %	14.27 %	7.9 %	9.25 %

Table 7.1: Volume exerted in consecutive heart beats.

In order to determine particle residence times, a stationary cutting mark is inserted into the geometry that separates atrium and ventricle along the MV plane at end-systole. Particles that leave the ventricle through the aorta are encapsulated by a forward LCS (blue in Figure 7.2). Particles which enter the ventricle through the cutting mark are enclosed by a backward LCS (red in Figure 7.2). The ejection fraction is altered in the post-processing to $EF = 42.09\,\%$, since the cutting mark is steady and the valve plane is moving. The resultant percentages of leaving blood volumes are listed in Table 7.1. Approximately 8 % of the blood particles leave the LV in the fourth beat and over 9 % are still located in the ventricle afterwards. These facts underline the incomplete ventricular washout.

Concluding, the vortex generation is physiological but the expected structures break down too early and are therefore lost during the systole. However, the washout and the maintenance of flow rotation are both expected to be enhanced if the outer resistant ring of the MV model comprises a larger area of the MV plane, whereby the blockage in the MV plane is increased. In other words, the effective opening area of the MV decreases and consequently the velocity of the entering blood jet is increased. Unfortunately, information on the patient-specific shape and size of the opening area in the MV plane is missing. This information should be included in future investigations. It can be obtained through projection of the patient-specific 3D valves onto the 2D valve plane during image processing of the MV (compare Chapter 6.4). Although the washout is not perfect, the overall results prove the applicability of the planar model realised via a moving porous media in an ALE framework.

8 Conclusion and Outlook

The identification of possible pathways to simplify *in-silico* heart flow models in comparison to the physiological human heart is the main objective of the present work. Thereby, the flow in the left side of the heart is in the centre of the investigation, since the LV has a higher potential to experience heart failure or valve diseases. Thus, the valve that is to be modelled is the MV, as it determines the inflow of the blood into the LV. Two major steps have been undertaken to achieve the defined goal. Firstly, reliable and meaningful post-processing techniques have been identified and characterised. Secondly, the role of the adopted valve model in the ventricle has been investigated and described. Particular focus has been posed in the vortex generation process as it represents the dominant flow characteristics in the human heart. Vortex generation and propagation, regions of dominating strain, cause-effect relations, mixing processes and particle residence times are quantities that are of special interest when the health status of a patient is to be classified. Therefore, the identification of the characteristics has to be credible.

Two methods have been chosen for vortex identification: the Q-criterion that locally detects regions of dominating flow rotation and the extraction of LCS that mark repelling and attracting material surfaces. With the choice of these two techniques a wide range of information can be gathered. The Q-criterion captures vortex generation at the MV, its detachment from the valve plane and its propagation into the ventricle. Further, the criterion serves as an indicator for regions where the local strain dominates over the flow rotation. Those regions are particularly relevant in blood flow dynamics, as blood cells can experience severe damage when they are exposed to stretching. The performed variation of the flow field resolution shows that it is not critical for a successful and reliable application of the Q-criterion. Unfortunately, a meaningful value for visualising the iso-surfaces of Q and thus vortex boundary detection is not available. Future work should continue first attempts to relate Q to other characteristic flow quantities and thereby identify globally applicable critical values.

Cause-effect relations are one feature that is better identified by LCS. Hereby, tracking particles forward in time highlights which volume portions will have the same dynamics within the next heart beat. Tracking particles backward in time reveals which volume portions had the same dynamics during the previous integration interval. Vortex boundaries and shear layers are located on the surfaces of the highest particle separation rate which corresponds to maxima in the FTLE field. If the surface is breaking apart, mixing of the two neighboured domains takes place. Further, the volumes of the wrapped particles within the LV enable the determination of particle residence times.

The FTLE result is dependent on the resolution of the velocity field in space and time and the number of seeded particles. It has been shown in the present thesis that all quantities interact with each other. Based on these findings, two criteria have been developed that allow the judgement of the resolution. Firstly, the sum criterion characterises the level of the spatial particle resolution, PP. If PP is too small, the FTLE field is coarse and thus the extracted LCS become poor in detail, making the flow structure indistinguishable. With the assumption that the FTLE is limited, the sum over all FTLE values strives towards an upper bound, which is directly linked to the spatial refinement rate. Secondly, the relative error criterion characterises the level of spatial resolution of the underlying velocity field, VP. This enables the local comparison of FTLE fields with different velocity grid resolutions. LCS extracted from an insufficient resolution preserve their sharpness but loose their proper positioning. A sufficiently fine resolution is reached if the relative error tends towards zero. The temporal resolution of the underlying velocity field, TP, determines if a Lagrangian particle tracking is possible. If the resolution is too coarse, the particles follow paths that are quasi streamlines and thus the LCS resemble Eulerian information. Both developed criteria show a transition zone between Eulerian and Lagrangian regime. It is important to detect the border resolution of the transition zone in order to judge whether the resolution in use lies in the Lagrangian regime. Since TP has the same effect on the results as VP, the relative error shows better performance compared to the sum criterion.

Investigation of the reciprocal influences of the spatial and temporal resolutions has shown that especially a combination of coarsening the spatial and temporal resolution of the underlying velocity data leads to wrongly located and shaped LCS. Then again, the particle resolution is nearly independent upon the underlying problem and data. It is primarily responsible for a sharp representation of the results. A generally applicable absolute value of sufficient resolution cannot be given, as it further depends on parameters such as the integration length. In the present work, the best cost-benefit relation for the LV has been achieved with $PP = 23$, $VP = 23$ with respect to the MV diameter as characteristic length scale and $TP = 100$ with respect to the duration of one heart beat as characteristic time scale. Future work will concentrate on the generalisation of such criteria for any flow problem. Knowing these numbers beforehand significantly accelerates the post-processing.

For the simulation of the heart flow, the validity of three common simplifications have been evaluated. Firstly, assuming a Newtonian fluid yields results comparable to clinical evidence with the advantage of reducing computational costs. However, the influence of inexpensive non-Newtonian models on the quality of the flow field cannot be reliably estimated, because they are trimmed for specific applications and comparable information for patient specific cases are missing. Secondly, it is not possible to describe the transition between a laminar and a turbulent flow with reasonable computational effort. A laminar solver is recommended over a turbulence model, as the flow in the LV is mostly laminar and only experiences transition locally and for a short time. Lastly, trabeculae and papillary muscles have been neglected in this work. Justification for this decision lies in the fact that measures such as residence times or the overall energy balance are not significantly affected and currently available imaging techniques do not provide adequate temporal and spatial resolutions.

Reviewing the literature, two MV models seem superior over the others, the planar MV model, thanks to its flexibility and ease of use, and the FSI MV model, as it is the closest to the physiological valve and provides additional information on the valve mechanics. Since only the flow in the LV is investigated in this work, the planar MV model and a 3D geometry-prescribed MV have been implemented and characterised. The shape of the utilised LV and atrium are idealised. While the atrium is assumed to be rigid, the ventricular wall movement is prescribed.

Evaluation of the flexibility of the planar MV model has shown that a variation of the valve orientation does not influence the particle residence time in the LV. Differences in the flow patterns are visible, yet only marginally, while the overall flow characteristics are not altered. Concluding, the results of the Q-criterion and the FTLE reveal physiological flow characteristics and prove the working concept of the planar MV model. In contrast, a simplification of the model into a diode type model has a visible and measurable impact on the mixing of the blood, particle residence times and vortex formation.

With the 3D geometry-prescribed MV, the detected structures in terms of Q-criterion and LCS extraction show less sharp borders, which suggests enhanced mixing. Quantitative comparison of the particle residence times of the 3D valve and its projection by means of the planar MV model has yielded that the expected optimisation of the ventricular washout is less than suggested by other studies. Both models produce physiological flow characteristics, i.e. a ring vortex forms at the MV, detaches during the diastole and tilts into the apex while travelling downwards in the LV. Future development has to include code optimisation, especially for the 3D MV model which is realised within an IBM framework. However, the ALE configuration with the planar MV is significantly faster. Currently, the calculation times differ by a factor of 20 and even with the suggested optimisations, the ALE seems to outperform the IBM. Additionally, a time-dependent projection of the effective opening area from a patient specific geometry is easier to generate and easier to implement compared to the reconstruction of a 3D MV. As such, the planar model outclasses the other in flexibility, handling and simulation time.

Finally, the applicability of the simple MV model in a patient specific framework has been proven. Therefore, the MV model has been implemented into a geometry much closer to clinical application than the idealised LV used for testing. This increased proximity to physiological conditions is accompanied by additional numerical challenges, i.e. increasing geometry complexity, enhanced mesh motion and a moving valve plane. The description of the porous valve plane has been altered from a Darcy-Forchheimer formulation to a forcing model that mimics moving mass in the porous zones. First results show the typical vortex formation and realistic particle residence times.

These results build a first step towards feasibility of heart flow simulations in the daily medical routine. As such, they have to be validated by comparison to experimental results or patient-specific flow measurement data. With respect to the clinical application, optimised cost-benefit strategies are of major interest. Thus, automation of the processes plays an important role in future research. Therein, the generation of the models, the simulation itself and the post-processing have to be included. In terms of the MV model, automation of the opening and closing in dependency of pressure differences or volume fluxes is the scope of the investigation following the present work.

Bibliography

[1] M. Al-Atabi, D. M. Espino, and D. W. Hukins. Computer and experimental modelling of blood flow through the mitral valve of the heart. *J Biomech Sci Eng*, 5(1):78–84, 2010.

[2] M. G. Al-Azawy, A. Turan, and A. Revell. Assessment of turbulence models for pulsatile flow inside a heart pump. *Comput Methods Biomech Biomed Engin*, 19(3):271–285, 2016. PMID: 25816074.

[3] A. Amblard, H. W.-L. Berre, B. Bou-Saïd, and M. Brunet. Analysis of type I endoleaks in a stented abdominal aortic aneurysm. *Med Eng Phys*, 31(1):27–33, 2009.

[4] J. B. Askov, J. L. Honge, M. O. Jensen, H. Nygaard, J. M. Hasenkam, and S. L. Nielsen. Significance of force transfer in mitral valve–left ventricular interaction: In vivo assessment. *J Thorac Cardiovasc Surg*, 145(6):1635 – 1641, 2013.

[5] M. Astorino, J. Hamers, S. C. Shadden, and J. F. Gerbeau. A robust and efficient valve model based on resistive immersed surfaces. *Int J Numer Method Biomed Eng*, 28(9):937–959, 2012.

[6] Aviva.co.uk. Medical encyclopedia - Function: How the heart beats. `https://www.aviva.co.uk/health-insurance/home-of-health/medical-centre/medical-encyclopedia`, 2017. Accessed: September 2017.

[7] B. Baccani, F. Domenichini, and G. Pedrizzetti. Model and influence of mitral valve opening during the left ventricular filling. *J Biomech*, 36(3):355 – 361, 2003.

[8] A. M. Bavo, A. M. Pouch, J. Degroote, J. Vierendeels, J. H. Gorman, R. C. Gorman, and P. Segers. Patient-specific CFD simulation of intraventricular haemodynamics based on 3d ultrasound imaging. *Biomed Eng Online*, 15(1):107, Sept. 2016.

[9] H. Binous. Introducing non-Newtonian fluid mechanics computations with Mathematica in the undergraduate curriculum. *Chem Eng Educ*, Winter Issue:59–64, 2007.

[10] Blausen.com staff. Medical gallery of Blausen Medical 2014. *WikiJournal of Medicine*, 1(2), 2014.

[11] I. Borazjani, J. Westerdale, E. M. McMahon, P. K. Rajaraman, J. J. Heys, and M. Belohlavek. Left ventricular flow analysis: Recent advances in numerical methods and applications in cardiac ultrasound. *Comput Math Methods Med*, 2013:11, 2013.

[12] M. Breuer. Numerische Strömungsmechanik. University lecture at Helmut-Schmidt-Universität Hamburg, March 2017.

[13] P. Cardiff, A. Karač, and A. Ivanković. A large strain finite volume method for orthotropic bodies with general material orientations. *Comput Methods Appl Mech Eng*, 268:318–335, 2014.

[14] P. J. Carreau. Rheological equations from molecular network theories. *Trans Soc Rheol*, 16(1):99–127, 1972.

[15] C. Chnafa, S. Mendez, and F. Nicoud. Image-based large-eddy simulation in a realistic left heart. *Comput Fluids*, 94:173–187, May 2014.

[16] Y. J. Choi, V. Vedula, and R. Mittal. Computational study of the dynamics of a bileaflet mechanical heart valve in the mitral position. *Ann Biomed Eng*, 42(8):1668–1680, 2014.

[17] S. K. Dahl, J. Vierendeels, J. Degroote, S. Annerel, L. R. Hellevik, and B. Skallerud. FSI simulation of asymmetric mitral valve dynamics during diastolic filling. *Comput Method Biomec*, 15(2):121–130, 2012.

[18] J. De Hart, G. Peters, G. Schreurs, and F. Baaijens. A two-dimensional fluid-structure interaction model of the aortic value. *J Biomech*, 33(9):1079–1088, 2000.

[19] J. Degroote, R. Haelterman, S. Annerel, P. Bruggeman, and J. Vierendeels. Performance of partitioned procedures in fluid-structure interaction. *Comput Struct*, 88(7):446 – 457, 2010.

[20] I. Demirdžić and M. Perić. Space conservation law in finite volume calculations of fluid flow. *International journal for numerical methods in fluids*, 8(9):1037–1050, 1988.

[21] F. Domenichini, G. Pedrizzetti, and B. Baccani. Three-dimensional filling flow into a model left ventricle. *J Fluid Mech*, 539:179–198, 2005.

[22] K. Dumont, J. Vierendeels, R. Kaminsky, G. Van Nooten, P. Verdonck, and D. Bluestein. Comparison of the hemodynamic and thrombogenic performance of two bileaflet mechanical heart valves using a CFD/FSI model. *J Biomech Eng*, 129(4):558–565, 2007.

[23] J. Eriksson. *Quantification of 4D Left Ventricular Blood Flow in Health and Disease*. PhD thesis, Linköping University, Sweden, 2013.

[24] D. M. Espino, D. E. Shepherd, and D. W. Hukins. Evaluation of a transient, simultaneous, arbitrary Lagrange-Euler based multi-physics method for simulating the mitral heart valve. *Comput Method Biomec*, 17(4):450–458, 2014.

[25] J. H. Ferziger and M. Perić. *Numerische Strömungsmechanik*. Springer Berlin Heidelberg, 2008.

[26] T. Fritz, C. Wieners, G. Seemann, H. Steen, and O. Dössel. Simulation of the contraction of the ventricles in a human heart model including atria and pericardium. *Biomech Model Mechanobiol*, 13(3):627–641, Jun 2014.

[27] R. Fuchs, R. Peikert, F. Sadlo, B. Alsallakh, and M. E. Gröller. Delocalized unsteady vortex region detectors. In *Vision, Modeling, and Visualization*, 2008.

[28] C. Garth, F. Gerhardt, X. Tricoche, and H. Hagen. Efficient computation and visualization of coherent structures in fluid flow applications. *IEEE Trans Vis Comput Graphics*, 13(6):1464–1471, 2007.

[29] F. Gijsen, E. Allanic, F. van de Vosse, and J. Janssen. The influence of the non-Newtonian properties of blood on the flow in large arteries: Unsteady flow in a 90° curved tube. *J Biomech*, 32(7):705 – 713, 1999.

[30] F. Gijsen, F. van de Vosse, and J. Janssen. The influence of the non-Newtonian properties of blood on the flow in large arteries: Steady flow in a carotid bifurcation model. *J Biomech*, 32(6):601 – 608, 1999.

[31] L. Goubergrits. Charité - Universitätsmedizin Berlin, personal communication, October 2016.

[32] L. Graftieaux, M. Michard, and N. Grosjean. Combining PIV, POD and vortex identification algorithms for the study of unsteady turbulent swirling flows. *Measurement Science and Technology*, 12(9):1422, 2001.

[33] C. J. Greenshields. Openfoam user guide. *OpenFOAM Foundation Ltd, version*, 3(1), 2015.

[34] G. Haller. An objective definition of a vortex. *J Fluid Mech*, 525:1–26, 2005.

[35] G. Haller. A variational theory of hyperbolic Lagrangian coherent structures. *Physica D*, 240(7):574–598, 2011.

[36] C. S. Harrison and G. A. Glatzmaier. Lagrangian coherent structures in the California current system–sensitivities and limitations. *Geophys Astro Fluid*, 106(1):22–44, 2012.

[37] R. B. Hinton and K. E. Yutzey. Heart valve structure and function in development and disease. *Annu Rev Physiol*, 73:29–46, 2011.

[38] G. Hou, J. Wang, and A. Layton. Numerical methods for fluid-structure interaction – A review. *Commun Comput Phys*, 12(2):337–377, 008 2012.

[39] J. Hron and S. Turek. *A Monolithic FEM/Multigrid Solver for an ALE Formulation of Fluid-Structure Interaction with Applications in Biomechanics*, pages 146–170. Springer Berlin Heidelberg, Berlin, Heidelberg, 2006.

[40] J. C. Hunt, A. Wray, and P. Moin. Eddies, streams, and convergence zones in turbulent flows. In *Studying Turbulence Using Numerical Simulation Databases, 2*, volume 1, pages 193–208, 1988.

[41] P. A. Iaizzo. *Handbook of cardiac anatomy, physiology, and devices*. Springer Science & Business Media, 2009.

[42] S. R. Idelsohn, F. Del Pin, R. Rossi, and E. Oñate. Fluid-structure interaction problems with strong added-mass effect. *Int J Numer Meth Eng*, 80(10):1261–1294, 2009.

[43] S. Irmay. On the theoretical derivation of Darcy and Forchheimer formulas. *EOS, Trans Am Geophys Union*, 39(4):702–707, 1958.

[44] H. Jasak. Dynamic mesh handling in OpenFOAM. In *Aerospace Sciences Meetings*, pages –. American Institute of Aeronautics and Astronautics, January 2009.

[45] D. Jospeh and B. Yang. Friction Factor Correlations for Laminar, Transition and Turbulent Flow in Smooth Pipes. *Physica D*, 239, 2010.

[46] F. Kaiser, A. Feldhusen, B. Roidl, M. Klaas, and J. Kriegseis. Lagrangian characterization of buffet-induced flow separation – A comparative analysis of tomographic-PIV and LES data. In *Proceedings der*

23. GALA-Fachtagung "Lasermethoden in der Strömungsmesstechnik", Dresden, Germany, September 8 - 10, 2015.

[47] H. Kantz. A robust method to estimate the maximal Lyapunov exponent of a time series. *Phys Lett A*, 185(1):77–87, 1994.

[48] S. Krittian. *Modellierung der kardialen Strömung-Struktur-Wechselwirkung*. PhD thesis, Karlsruhe Institute of Technology (KIT), 2009.

[49] S. Krittian, T. Schenkel, U. Janoske, and H. Oertel. Partitioned fluid-solid coupling for cardiovascular blood flow: Validation study of pressure-driven fluid-domain deformation. *Ann Biomed Eng*, 38(8):2676–2689, 2010.

[50] K. Kunzelman, D. R. Einstein, and R. Cochran. Fluid–structure interaction models of the mitral valve: Function in normal and pathological states. *Phil Trans R Soc B*, 362(1484):1393–1406, 2007.

[51] U. Küttler and W. A. Wall. Fixed-point fluid-structure interaction solvers with dynamic relaxation. *Comput Mech*, 43(1):61–72, 2008.

[52] D. Larsson, J. H. Spühler, E. Günyeli, T. Weinkauf, J. Hoffman, M. Colarieti-Tosti, R. Winter, and M. Larsson. Estimation of left ventricular blood flow parameters–clinical application of patient-specific CFD simulations from 4d echocardiography. In *SPIE Medical Imaging*, pages 101390L–101390L. International Society for Optics and Photonics, 2017.

[53] T. B. Le and F. Sotiropoulos. On the three-dimensional vortical structure of early diastolic flow in a patient-specific left ventricle. *Eur J Mech B-Fluid*, 35(0):20–24, Sept. 2012.

[54] J. D. Lemmon and A. P. Yoganathan. Computational modeling of left heart diastolic function: Examination of ventricular dysfunction. *J Biomech Eng*, 122(4):297–303, 2000.

[55] J. D. Lemmon and A. P. Yoganathan. Three-dimensional computational model of left heart diastolic function with fluid-structure interaction. *J Biomech Eng*, 122(2):109–117, 2000.

[56] Q. Long, R. Merrifield, X. Xu, P. Kilner, D. Firmin, and G. Yang. Subject-specific computational simulation of left ventricular flow based on magnetic resonance imaging. *Proc Inst Mech Eng H*, 222(4):475–485, 2008.

[57] J. O. Mangual, F. Domenichini, and G. Pedrizzetti. Describing the highly three dimensional right ventricle flow. *Ann Biomed Eng*, 40(8):1790–1801, 2012.

[58] The Mathworks, Inc., Natick, Massachusetts. *MATLAB version 9.2.0.538062 (R2017a)*, 2017.

[59] D. M. McQueen and C. S. Peskin. A three-dimensional computer model of the human heart for studying cardiac fluid dynamics. *SIGGRAPH Comput Graph*, 34(1):56–60, Feb. 2000.

[60] V. Mihalef, R. I. Ionasec, P. Sharma, B. Georgescu, I. Voigt, M. Suehling, and D. Comaniciu. Patient-specific modelling of whole heart anatomy, dynamics and haemodynamics from four-dimensional cardiac CT images. *Interface Focus*, 1(3):286–296, 2011.

[61] R. Mittal and G. Iaccarino;. Immersed boundary methods. *Annu Rev Fluid Mech*, 37:239–61, 2005.

[62] R. D. Moser, J. Kim, and N. N. Mansour. Direct numerical simulation of turbulent channel flow up to Re_τ=590. *Phys Fluids*, 11(4), 1999.

[63] M.-P. Mühlhausen. *Strömung-struktur-gekoppelte Modellierung und Simulation des menschlichen Herzens*. PhD thesis, Karlsruhe, KIT, 2012.

[64] T. Mullin and J. Peixinho. Transition to turbulence in pipe flow. *J Low Temp Phys*, 145, 2006.

[65] M. Nakamura, S. Wada, T. Mikami, A. Kitabatake, and T. Karino. A computational fluid mechanical study on the effects of opening and closing of the mitral orifice on a transmitral flow velocity profile and an early diastolic intraventricular flow. *JSME Int J C Mech Sy*, 45(4):913–922, 2002.

[66] M. Nakamura, S. Wada, and T. Yamaguchi. Influence of the opening mode of the mitral valve orifice on intraventricular hemodynamics. *Ann Biomed Eng*, 34(6):927–935, 2006.

[67] D. Nordsletten, P. Hunter, and N. Smith. Conservative and non-conservative arbitrary Lagrangian–Eulerian forms for ventricular flows. *Int J Numer Meth Fluids*, 56(8):1457–1463, 2008.

[68] D. Nordsletten, M. McCormick, P. J. Kilner, P. Hunter, D. Kay, and N. P. Smith. Fluid-solid coupling for the investigation of diastolic and systolic human left ventricular function. *Int J Numer Method Biomed Eng*, 27(7):1017–1039, 2010.

[69] H. Oertel and S. B. S. Krittian. *Modelling the human cardiac fluid mechanics, 4. ed.* KIT Scientific Publishing, Karlsruhe, 2012.

[70] A. B. Olcay, T. S. Pottebaum, and P. S. Krueger. Sensitivity of Lagrangian coherent structure identification to flow field resolution and random errors. *Chaos*, 20(1):017506, 2010.

[71] G. Pedrizzetti and F. Domenichini. Nature optimizes the swirling flow in the human left ventricle. *Phys Rev Lett*, 95:108101, Sep 2005.

[72] M. Perschall. *Numerische Untersuchung des Wellenpumpenkonzeptes und der mechanischen HerzunterstÃ¼tzung*. PhD thesis, Karlsruhe Institute of Technology (KIT), 2010.

[73] C. S. Peskin. The immersed boundary method. *Acta Numer*, 11(0):479–517, 2002.

[74] C. S. Peskin and D. M. McQueen. A three-dimensional computational method for blood flow in the heart I. Immersed elastic fibers in a viscous incompressible fluid. *J Comput Phys*, 81(2):372 – 405, 1989.

[75] M. Reik, G. Meyrowitz, M. Schwarz, S. Donisi, T. Schenkel, and U. Kiencke. A 1d circulation model as boundary condition for a 3d simulation of a pumping human ventricle. In *IFMBE Proceedings*, volume 11, 2005.

[76] D. E. Rival, J. Kriegseis, P. Schaub, A. Widmann, and C. Tropea. Characteristic length scales for vortex detachment on plunging profiles with varying leading-edge geometry. *Exp Fluids*, 55(1):1660, 2014.

[77] N. R. Saber, N. B. Wood, A. D. Gosman, R. D. Merrifield, G.-Z. Yang, C. L. Charrier, P. D. Gatehouse, and D. N. Firmin. Progress towards patient-specific computational flow modeling of the left heart via combination of magnetic resonance imaging with computational fluid dynamics. *Ann Biomed Eng*, 31(1):42–52, 2003.

[78] A. Sadarjoen and F. H. Post. Detection, quantification, and tracking of vortices using streamline geometry. *Comput Graph*, 24(3):333–341, 2000.

[79] F. Sadlo and R. Peikert. Efficient visualization of Lagrangian coherent structures by filtered AMR ridge extraction. *IEEE Trans Vis Comput Graphics*, 13(6):1456–1463, Nov.-Dec. 2007.

[80] T. Schenkel, M. Malve, M. Reik, M. Markl, B. Jung, and H. Oertel. MRI-based CFD analysis of flow in a human left ventricle: Methodology and application to a healthy heart. *Ann Biomed Eng*, 37(3):503–515, 2009.

[81] B. Schindler, R. Peikert, R. Fuchs, and H. Theisel. Ridge concepts for the visualization of Lagrangian coherent structures. In *Topological Methods in Data Analysis and Visualization II*, pages 221–235. Springer, 2012.

[82] H. Schlichting. *Boundary-layer theory*, volume 7. McGraw-Hill Book Company, New York, 1979.

[83] H. Schlichting and K. Gersten. *Grenzschichttheorie*. Springer, 2005.

[84] P. P. Sengupta, G. Pedrizzetti, P. J. Kilner, A. Kheradvar, T. Ebbers, G. Tonti, A. G. Fraser, and J. Narula. Emerging trends in CV flow visualization. *JACC Cardiovasc Imaging*, 5(3):305–316, 2012.

[85] J. H. Seo and R. Mittal. Effect of diastolic flow patterns on the function of the left ventricle. *Phys Fluids*, 25(11):110801, 2013.

[86] J. H. Seo, V. Vedula, T. Abraham, A. C. Lardo, F. Dawoud, H. Luo, and R. Mittal. Effect of the mitral valve on diastolic flow patterns. *Phys Fluids*, 26(12):121901, 2014.

[87] S. Shadden. *Transport and Mixing in Laminar Flows*, chapter Lagrangian Coherent Structures, pages 59–89. Wiley-VCH Verlag GmbH & Co. KGaA, 2011.

[88] S. C. Shadden, J. O. Dabiri, and J. E. Marsden. Lagrangian analysis of fluid transport in empirical vortex ring flows. *Phys Fluids*, 18(4), 2006.

[89] S. C. Shadden, F. Lekien, and J. E. Marsden. Definition and properties of Lagrangian coherent structures from finite-time Lyapunov exponents in two-dimensional aperiodic flows. *Physica D*, 212(3):271–304, 2005.

[90] S. C. Shadden, F. Lekien, J. D. Paduan, F. P. Chavez, and J. E. Marsden. The correlation between surface drifters and coherent structures based on high-frequency radar data in Monterey bay. *Deep -Sea Res Pt II*, 56(3):161–172, 2009.

[91] F. Sotiropoulos and I. Borazjani. A review of state-of-the-art numerical methods for simulating flow through mechanical heart valves. *Med Biol Eng Comput*, 47(3):245–256, 2009.

[92] K. Spiegel. *Strömungsmechanischer Beitrag zur Planung von Herzoperationen*. PhD thesis, Karlsruhe Institute of Technology (KIT), 2009.

[93] J. H. Spurk and N. Aksel. *Strömungslehre: Einführung in die Theorie der Strömungen*. Springer Berlin Heidelberg, 2010.

[94] J. Stijnen, A. Bogaerds, J. de Hart, P. Bovendeerd, B. de Mol, and F. van de Vosse. Computational analysis of ventricular valve–valve interaction: Influence of flow conditions. *Int J Comut Fluid Dyn*, 23(8):609–622, 2009.

[95] M. Tabor and I. Klapper. Stretching and alignment in chaotic and turbulent flows. *Chaos, Solitons Fractals*, 4(6):1031 – 1055, 1994. Special Issue: Chaos Applied to Fluid Mixing.

[96] P. L. Tallec and J. Mouro. Fluid structure interaction with large structural displacements. *Comput Methods in Appl Mech Eng*, 190(24):3039 – 3067, 2001.

[97] N. P. Thien and R. I. Tanner. A new constitutive equation derived from network theory. *J Non-Newton Fluid*, 2(4):353–365, 1977.

[98] Ž. Tuković and H. Jasak. Updated Lagrangian finite volume solver for large deformation dynamic response of elastic body. *T FAMENA*, 31(1):55, 2007.

[99] Ž. Tuković and H. Jasak. Immersed boundary method in OpenFOAM. In *7th OpenFOAM® Workshop, Technische Universität Darmstadt, Germany*, pages 25–28, 2012.

[100] S. Turek and J. Hron. Proposal for numerical benchmarking of fluid-structure interaction between an elastic object and laminar incompressible flow. In H.-J. Bungartz and M. Schäfer, editors, *Lecture Notes in Computational Science and Engineering*, volume 53, pages 371–385. Springer Berlin Heidelberg, 2006.

[101] S. Uchida. The pulsating viscous flow superposed on the steady laminar motion of incompressible fluid in a circular pipe. *ZAMP*, 7(5):403–422, 1956.

[102] V. Vedula, S. Fortini, J. H. Seo, G. Querzoli, and R. Mittal. Computational modeling and validation of intraventricular flow in a simple model of the left ventricle. *Theor Comp Fluid Dyn*, 28(6):589–604, 2014.

[103] V. Vedula, J.-H. Seo, A. C. Lardo, and R. Mittal. Effect of trabeculae and papillary muscles on the hemodynamics of the left ventricle. *Theor Comp Fluid Dyn*, 30(1):3–21, 2016.

[104] J. Vierendeels, K. R. ans E Dick, and P. Verdonck. Computer simulation of intraventricular flow and pressure gradients during diastole. *J Biomech Eng*, 122(6)(0148-0731 (Linking)):667–74, 2000.

[105] D. K. Walters and D. Cokljat. A three equation eddy-viscosity model for Reynolds-averaged Navier-Stokes simulations of transitional flow. *J Fluids Eng*, 130(12):121401, 2008.

[106] D. K. Walters and J. H. Leylek. A new model for boundary layer transition using a single-point RANS approach. *J Turbomach*, 126, 2004.

[107] L. Wang, L.-P. Wang, Z. Guo, and J. Mi. Volume-averaged macroscopic equation for fluid flow in moving porous media. *Int J Heat Mass Transf*, 82:357–368, 2015.

[108] S. b. Wang, L. Lee, and J. Lee. A linear relation between the compressibility and density of blood. *J Acoust Soc Am*, 109(1):390–396, 2001. cited By 27.

[109] H. Watanabe, T. Hisada, S. Sugiura, J.-i. Okada, and H. Fukunari. Computer simulation of blood flow, left ventricular wall motion and their interrelationship by fluid-structure interaction finite element method. *JSME Int J C Mech Sy*, 45(4):1003–1012, 2002.

[110] H. Watanabe, S. Sugiura, H. Kafuku, and T. Hisada. Multiphysics simulation of left ventricular filling dynamics using fluid-structure interaction finite element method. *Biophys J*, 87(3):2074 – 2085, 2004.

[111] S. Whitaker. Flow in porous media I: A theoretical derivation of Darcy's law. *Transport Porous Med*, 1(1):3–25, 1986.

[112] WHO. *World health statistics 2015*. World Health Organization, 2015.

[113] A. Willis, J. Peixinho, R. Kerswell, and T. Mulllin. Experimental and theoretical progress in pipe flow transition. *Phil Trans R Soc A*, 366, 2008.

[114] T. Ye, R. Mittal, H. Udaykumar, and W. Shyy. An accurate Cartesian grid method for viscous incompressible flows with complex immersed boundaries. *J Comput Phys*, 156(2):209–240, 1999.

[115] B. M. Yun, L. P. Dasi, C. K. Aidun, and A. P. Yoganathan. Highly resolved pulsatile flows through prosthetic heart valves using the entropic lattice-Boltzmann method. *J Fluid Mech*, 754:122–160, 2014.

[116] Y. Zhang, K. Liu, H. Xian, and X. Du. A review of methods for vortex identification in hydroturbines. *Renew Sus Energ Rev*, 2017.

Conference Contributions and Publications

[DFK16] A. Daub, B. Frohnapfel, and J. Kriegseis. Left ventricular flow field evaluation - A step toward generalization of post-processing techniques. 87th Annu Meeting Int Assoc Appl Mathematics and Mechanics, Braunschweig, Germany, March 8 2016.

[DKF16] A. Daub, J. Kriegseis, and B. Frohnapfel. Sensitivity analysis of a three plane diode type mitral valve model. 11th Eur Fluid Mechanics Conf, Seville, Spain, September 15 2016.

[SGK+15] A. Slotosch, M. Gollub, F. Kaiser, B. Frohnapfel, and J. Kriegseis. Lagrangian coherent structures in unsteady flow fields – Required resolution of the field information. In *Proceedings der 23. GALA-Fachtagung "Lasermethoden in der Strömungsmesstechnik", Dresden, Germany*, 2015.

[SKF15] A. Slotosch, J. Kriegseis, and B. Frohnapfel. Effect of different diode type mitral valve models on left ventricular flow pattern. BMES Annu Meeting, Tampa, USA, October 9 2015.

[SSKK14] A. Slotosch, J. Schlanderer, F. Kaiser, and J. Kriegseis. Heart flow vortices – An application of flow characterization techniques. In *Proceedings der 22. GALA-Fachtagung "Lasermethoden in der Strömungsmesstechnik", Karlsruhe, Germany*, 2014.

Co-Supervised Student Theses

If not otherwise stated the theses were conducted at the Karlsruhe Institute of Technology (KIT), Institute of Fluid Mechanics (ISTM).

Alkemper, F. (2017). *Untersuchung von Wandbewegungsmodellen zur Simulation von Herzströmungen*. Bachelor thesis.

Bakar, A. (2015). *Mitral Valve Simulation in Computational Fluid Dynamics*. Bachelor thesis.

Brakhage, J. (2016). *Examination of criteria to characterize an FTLE calculation*. Master thesis.

Gollub, M. (2013). *Weiterentwicklung der Fluid-Struktur-Interaktion in OpenFOAM um nichtnewtonsche Fluide und hyperelastische Materialien*. Bachelor thesis.

Gollub, M. (2015). *Charakterisierung eines Wirbelidentifikationstools zur effizienten FTLE-Berechnung*. Master thesis.

Hütter, L. (2016). *Untersuchung eines Herstellungsverfahrens für ein elastisches Modell des Aortenbogens für Particle Image Velocimetry (PIV) Messungen*. Bachelor thesis, in cooperation with University of Canterburry, Department of Mechanical Engineering.

Kaiser, F. (2014). *Heart Flow Vortices – an FTLE Approach*. Master thesis.

Klatt, J.-N. (2015). *Verification and Validation of a Three-Equation Transition Model for Application to Internal Flows*. Master thesis.

Meyer, D. (2014). *Weiterentwicklung der Fluid-Struktur-Interaktion in OpenFOAM*. Master thesis.

Schlanderer, J. (2014). *Heart Flow Vortices – Comparison of Vortex Detection Methods*. Bachelor thesis.

Stark, T. (2013). *Konzeptentwicklung zur Fluid-Struktur-Interaktion mit der Immersed Boundary Methode in OpenFOAM*. Bachelor thesis.

Vellguth, K. (2017). *Numerical Simulation of the Early Diastolic Left Ventricular Blood Flow*. Master thesis, in cooperation with Charité - Universitätsmedizin Berlin, Institute for Computational and Imaging Science in Cardiovascular Medicine.

Nomenclature

All indices used (i,j,k...) run from $1-3$. The superscript * indicates that the quantity is scaled to be dimensionless. The superscripts $^{-}$ and $'$ used with flow quantities indicate the time average and time-dependent fluctuation of the respective quantity. The superscript $^{+}$ marks quantities scaled in plus units.

Latin letters – Upper case

SYMBOL	SI UNIT	DESCRIPTION
A	$\mathrm{m^2\,s^{-1}}$	stream function constant
A_{BP}		model constant in bypass transition
$\mathbf{C}$		right Cauchy-Green tensor
$C_0 \ldots C_4$		constants
$C_{\omega 1\ldots 3}$, $C_{\omega R}$		model constants in ω transport equation
$C_{R,\mathrm{BP}}$, $C_{R,\mathrm{NAT}}$		coefficients in transition
D_l	$\mathrm{m^2\,s^{-2}}$	anisotropic laminar dissipation
D_T	$\mathrm{m^2\,s^{-2}}$	anisotropic turbulent dissipation
E	$\mathrm{kg\,m^{-1}\,s^{-2}}$	Young's modulus
EF	%	ejection fraction
F	$\mathrm{kg\,m\,s^{-2}}$	acting force

F_p	$\mathrm{kg\,m\,s^{-2}}$	porous media forcing term
L	m	channel length
L_c	m	characteristic length scale
L_V	m	ventricle length
N		total number of particles
P		centre point of stencil
P_{k_L}	$\mathrm{m^2\,s^{-2}}$	laminar kinetic energy production
P_{k_T}	$\mathrm{m^2\,s^{-2}}$	turbulent kinetic energy production
PP		particle points
Q		second invariant of the velocity gradient
Q'		strain rotation modified Q
R	m	radius
R_{BP}	$\mathrm{m^2\,s^{-3}}$	bypass transition term
Re		Reynolds number
Re_b		bulk Reynolds number
Re_τ		friction Reynolds number
R_{NAT}	$\mathrm{m^2\,s^{-3}}$	natural transition term
S_{ij}	$\mathrm{s^{-1}}$	strain rate tensor
St		Strouhal number
T_c	s	characteristic time scale
T_{int}	s	time integration interval
TP		time points
U_c	$\mathrm{m\,s^{-1}}$	characteristic velocity
U_{in}	$\mathrm{m\,s^{-1}}$	inlet velocity

U_{out}	$\mathrm{m\,s^{-1}}$	outlet velocity
V_{dia}	$\mathrm{m^3}$	end-diastolic volume
V_{stroke}	$\mathrm{m^3}$	stroke volume
V_{sys}	$\mathrm{m^3}$	end-systolic volume
$\dot{V}_{in}$	$\mathrm{m^3\,s^{-1}}$	in-going flow rate
VP		velocity points
Wo		Womersley number
W_{pV}	$\mathrm{m^5\,s^{-2}}$	pressure-volume work

Latin letters – Lower case

SYMBOL	SI UNIT	DESCRIPTION
a, b	m	lateral element displacement
c		stream function constant
c_i	$\mathrm{m\,s^{-1}}$	mesh velocity
d	m	pipe diameter
d_{MV}	m	mitral valve diameter
d_W	m	wall distance
f_D		Darcy friction factor
f_i	$\mathrm{kg\,m\,s^{-2}}$	volume force
f_W		wall damping function
h	m	half channel height
k	$\mathrm{m^2\,s^{-1}}$	mesh motion diffusivity
k_1		constant in restriction of Euclidean norm
k_p	$\mathrm{m^2}$	permeability

k_L	$m^2\,s^{-2}$	laminar kinetic energy
k_T	$m^2\,s^{-2}$	turbulent kinetic energy
l	m	length
m	kg	fluid mass
m_s	kg	solid mass
n		exponent in Carreau viscosity model
n_i, $\vec{n}$	m	boundary normal vector
p	$kg\,m^{-1}\,s^{-2}$	pressure
r	m	radial coordinate
t	s	time
u_b	$m\,s^{-1}$	bulk velocity
u_i	$m\,s^{-1}$	fluid velocity
u_τ		friction velocity
v_i	$m\,s^{-1}$	solid velocity
x	m	displacement
x', y'	m	local Cartesian coordinate
x_0	m	particle starting position
x_i	m	Cartesian coordinate
x_{rel}	m	relative distance
x_s	m	solid translation

Greek letters – Upper case

SYMBOL	SI UNIT	DESCRIPTION
Γ	m^2	boundary surface of geometry
Δt	s	time step size
$\Delta\Theta$	$^\circ$	angular displacement
Δx, Δy, Δz	m	grid spacing
Δx_1, Δx_2	m	edge lengths
ΔV	m^3	volume growth within time interval
$\Theta(x,y,t)$	$m^2\,s^{-1}$	analytical stream function
Φ		placeholder for arbitrary variable
$\Phi_{t_0}^{t_1}$	m	flow map
Ω	s^{-1}	magnitude of mean rotation rate tensor
Ω_f	m^3	internal fluid volume
Ω_s	m^3	external solid volume
Ω_{ij}	s^{-1}	rotation tensor
Ω'_{ij}	s^{-1}	rotation rate of the strain axes

Greek letters – Lower case

SYMBOL	SI UNIT	DESCRIPTION
α	$^\circ$	valve plane tilting angle
α_T	$m^2\,s^{-1}$	effective diffusivity
β	m^{-1}	Forchheimer coefficient
β_{BP}, β_{NAT}		threshold functions for transition
δx_0	m	infinitesimal distance

$\delta\Phi_{t_0}^{t_1}$	m	difference between two flow maps
ϵ	m	roughness height
ε		error in sum criterion
$\varepsilon(p)$		field of local relative FTLE error
$\hat{\varepsilon}$		median of $\epsilon\ (p)$
$\dot{\gamma}$	s^{-1}	shear rate
λ_f	s	material parameter of Carreau viscosity model
λ_{max}		largest eigenvalue of the Cauchy-Green tensor
μ	$kg\,m^{-1}\,s^{-1}$	dynamic viscosity
μ_0, μ_∞	$kg\,m^{-1}\,s^{-1}$	upper and lower viscosity limits
μ_{eff}	$kg\,m^{-1}\,s^{-1}$	effective dynamic viscosity
μ_s	$kg\,m^{-1}\,s^{-2}$	shear modulus
ν	$m^2\,s^{-1}$	kinematic viscosity
ν_s	$m^2\,s^{-1}$	Poisson ratio
ν_T	$m^2\,s^{-1}$	turbulent eddy viscosity
π		ratio of a circle's circumference to its diameter
ρ	$kg\,m^{-3}$	fluid density
ρ_s	$kg\,m^{-3}$	solid density
$\sigma_{ij,s}$	$kg\,m^{-1}\,s^{-2}$	surface forces per unit area
$\sigma_{t_0}^{t_1}$, σ_p	s^{-1}	finite-time Lyapunov exponent
$\bar{\sigma}$	s^{-1}	mean finite-time Lyapunov exponent
σ_k, σ_ω		turbulent transport constants
σ_{ref}	s^{-1}	reference finite-time Lyapunov exponent
τ	$kg\,m^{-1}\,s^{-2}$	shear stress

τ_{ij}	$\mathrm{kg\,m^{-1}\,s^{-2}}$	stress tensor
τ_w	$\mathrm{kg\,m^{-1}\,s^{-1}}$	wall shear stress
ϕ		random flow variable
$\bar{\phi}$		time averaged flow variable
ϕ'		time-dependent variable fluctuations
ϕ_p		porosity
ω	$\mathrm{s^{-1}}$	specific dissipation rate
ω_f	$\mathrm{s^{-1}}$	angular frequency
ω_i	$\mathrm{s^{-1}}$	vorticity vector

Mathematical operators

SYMBOL	DESCRIPTION
$\partial(\ldots)$	partial derivative
$\mathrm{d}(\ldots)$	total derivative
$\frac{\mathrm{D}(\ldots)}{\mathrm{D}t}$	material derivative
e	exponential function
ϵ_{ijk}	Levi-Cevita symbol
$\nabla(\ldots)$	gradient
$\iint\limits_A(\ldots)\mathrm{d}A$	surface integral
$\iiint\limits_V(\ldots)\mathrm{d}V$	volume integral
$\sum\limits_{i=1..N}(\ldots)$	sum of N elements with running index i
$\mathrm{tr}(\ldots)$	trace of a matrix

Abbreviations

SYMBOL	DESCRIPTION
1D	one-dimensional
2D	two-dimensional
3D	three-dimensional
ALE	arbitrary Lagrangian-Eulerian
CFL	Courant-Friedrich-Levi number
DNS	direct numerical simulation
FSI	fluid-structure interaction
FTLE	finite-time Lyapunov exponent
IB	immersed boundary
IBM	immersed boundary method
LA	left atrium
LCS	Lagrangian coherent structures
LV	left ventricle
MRI	magnetic resonance imaging
MV	mitral valve
NSE	Navier-Stokes equations
RANS	Reynolds averaged Navier-Stokes
VP_1	one valve plane
VP_3	three valve planes

List of Figures

List of Tables

A Appendix

A.1 Solver Settings

The solver settings used throughout this work are shortly presented and discussed in the following.

All simulations are carried out using the backward scheme for time discretisation [33]. It is a explicit second-order time scheme that shows stable performance in all cases and is chosen to guarantee the proper representation of the time evolution. An alternative with comparable accuracy is the Crank-Nicholson scheme In OpenFOAM it can be blended with the explicit first-order Euler scheme via an of-centring coefficient. The blending coefficient is regulated between zero – fully explicit – and one – pure Crank-Nicholson – where the latter is unstable in some cases [33]. For the cases discussed in this work, a factor of 0.9 has shown good stability while maintaining a high accuracy. It yields the same results as the backward scheme.

In simple cases without wall movement, the second-order Gauss linear scheme shows good performance in terms of gradient discretisation. When wall movement is included, the scheme tends to generate oscillating results, which is why the least squares method is chosen instead. The least squares gradient scheme is of second-order accuracy on tetrahedral as well as hexahedral meshes. It uses the weighted gradient of all neighbouring cells to construct the gradient at the current location. To prevent over- or under-shoots of the gradient, the scheme is limited by the values of the surrounding faces.

Although the Gauss upwind scheme is often not accurate, it has essential stabilising effects on the solver performance. Peaks in the solution of the convection term are reduced due to its smearing influence. Using a Gauss linear scheme instead has shown the oscillating nature of this scheme. Even a blending between the two, resulting in the Gauss linear-upwind scheme, resulted in oscillating solutions that lead to divergence of the solution process. A mesh refinement reduces the observed effects. Unfortunately, the finer the mesh, the more computational time has to be accepted. Further, if the large scale structures are of primary interest, a proper mesh refinement does not significantly alter the results.

The Laplace operator is discretised using the Gauss linear scheme with correction for non-orthogonal meshes.

Listing A.1: Solver settings for cases without wall movement.

```
*****************************************
ddtSchemes          backward;
gradSchemes         Gauss linear;
divSchemes          Gauss upwind;
laplacianSchemes    Gauss linear corrected;
*****************************************
```

Listing A.2: Solver settings for cases with wall movement.

```
********************************************
ddtSchemes          backward;
gradSchemes         faceLimited leastSquares 1;
divSchemes
        default     Gauss linear;
        div(phi,U)  Gauss upwind;
laplacianSchemes    Gauss linear limited 0.5;
********************************************
```

A.2 Vortex Detection – Von Kármán Vortex Street

Figure A.1 shows the contours of the Q-criterion and exemplary a backward LCS. It can be seen, how the Q-criterion identifies vortex cores within the slings of the LCS. Thereby, the LCS marks the boundaries of the corresponding vortices.

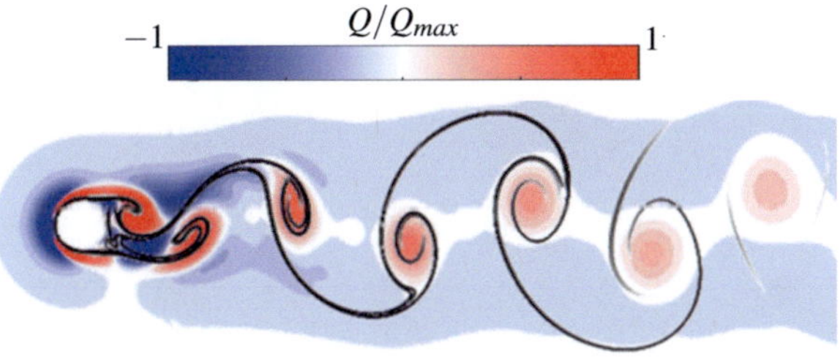

Figure A.1: Von Kármán vortex street: Q-criterion superimposed by an LCS determined by the backward FTLE.

Application of the error criteria for constant PP and VP and varying TP results in more fluctuating curve progressions in comparison to the evaluation of the double gyre flow (compare Figure A.3). As the von Kármán vortex street is an external flow, particles can leave the velocity area. The pathlines of the respective particles have to be interpolated. In this work, the velocity of particles leaving the area in either positive or negative x-direction is approximated by a constant velocity equal to the bulk velocity of the flow. Since this approximation does not fulfil the physical behaviour, errors are introduced for all FTLE evaluations. Furthermore, the vortices of the von Kármán vortex street occupy approximately one third of the whole evaluated flow field. As such, the region containing small FTLE values is significantly larger compared to the region of FTLE ridges. Application of the median error in case of the global relative error might therefore underestimate the actual error of the calculation.

Overall, Figure A.2 shows that combining the error criteria leads to a similar error distribution as in the case of the double gyre. As such, an ideal combination of sufficient fine resolutions at the lowest possible costs can be found at the crossing of the specified error bounds.

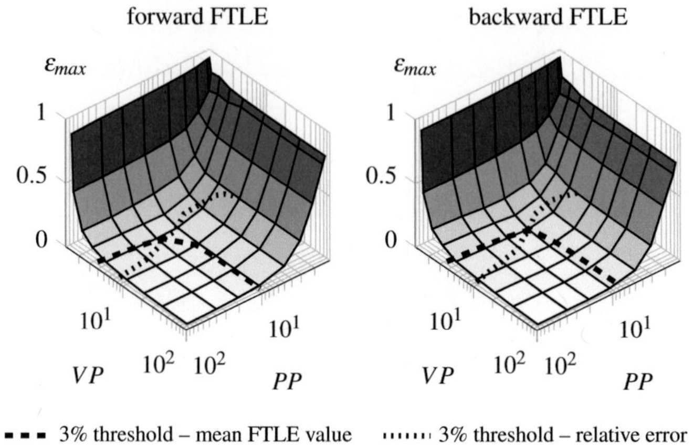

Figure A.2: Von Kármán vortex street: Combined global relative error and mean FTLE error for varying *PP* and *VP* at constant *TP* for (left) the forward FTLE and (right) the backward FTLE. The comparison is performed with the finest reference solution.

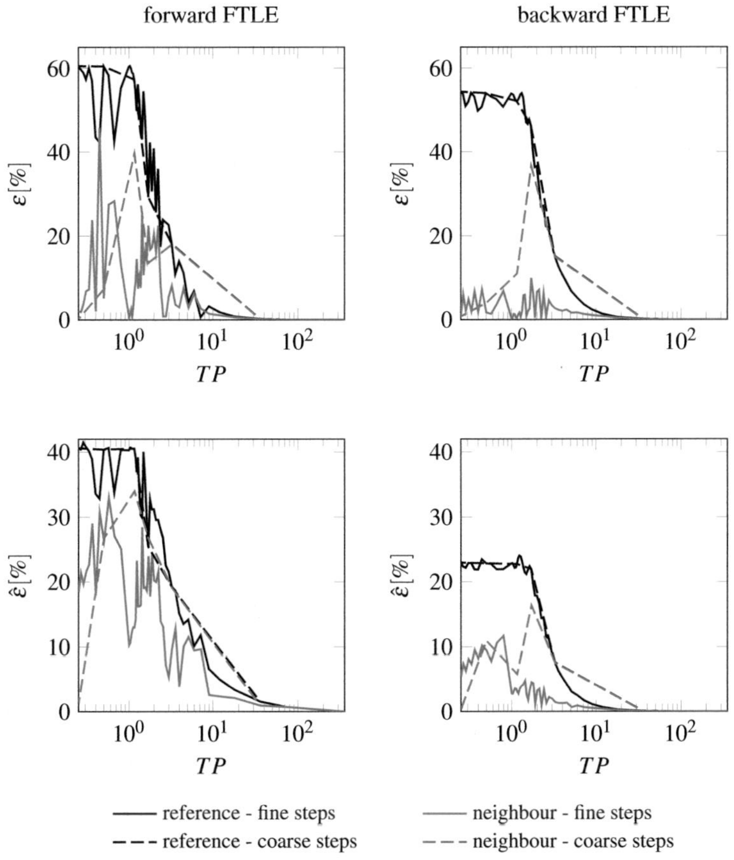

Figure A.3: Kármán vortex street: (top) Resulting error of the mean FTLE value and (bottom) resulting global relative error comparing the local FTLE value to either the finest reference solution or the finer neighbouring solution. Results are shown for (left) the forward FTLE and (right) the backward FTLE. TP is altered in coarse steps, ongoing doubled, or fine steps of $0.01TP$.

A.3 Details on the Transition Modelling

The transport equations for the turbulent kinetic energy, k_T, the laminar kinetic energy, k_L, and the specific dissipation rate, ω, are given by Walters and Cokljat [105], as

$$\begin{aligned}\frac{\mathrm{D}k_T}{\mathrm{D}t} = & \underbrace{P_{k_T}}_{production} \underbrace{+R_{\mathrm{BP}} + R_{\mathrm{NAT}}}_{transition} - \underbrace{\omega k_T}_{\substack{isotropic\\dissipation}} \\ & - \underbrace{D_T}_{\substack{anisotropic\\dissipation}} + \underbrace{\frac{\partial}{\partial x_j}\left[\left(\nu + \frac{\alpha_T}{\sigma_k}\right)\frac{\partial k_T}{\partial x_j}\right]}_{turbulent\ transport},\end{aligned} \tag{A.1}$$

$$\frac{\mathrm{D}k_L}{\mathrm{D}t} = \underbrace{P_{k_L}}_{production} \underbrace{-R_{\mathrm{BP}} - R_{\mathrm{NAT}}}_{transition} - \underbrace{D_l}_{\substack{anisotropic\\dissipation}} + \underbrace{\frac{\partial}{\partial x_j}\left[\nu\frac{\partial k_L}{\partial x_j}\right]}_{turbulent\ transport} \tag{A.2}$$

$$\begin{aligned}\frac{\mathrm{D}\omega}{\mathrm{D}t} = & \underbrace{C_{\omega 1}\frac{\omega}{k_T}P_{k_T}}_{production} + \underbrace{\left(\frac{C_{\omega R}}{f_W} - 1\right)\frac{\omega}{k_T}(R_{\mathrm{BP}} + R_{\mathrm{NAT}})}_{transition\ production} - \underbrace{C_{\omega 2}\omega^2}_{dissipation}, \\ & + \underbrace{C_{\omega 3} f_\omega \alpha_T f_W^2 \frac{\sqrt{k_T}}{d_W^3}}_{boundary\ layer\ wake\ term} + \underbrace{\frac{\partial}{\partial x_j}\left[\left(\nu + \frac{\alpha_T}{\sigma_\omega}\right)\frac{\partial \omega}{\partial x_j}\right]}_{turbulent\ transport}.\end{aligned} \tag{A.3}$$

Alike other RANS models, the equations include terms for energy production, dissipation and transportation. In terms of the transition process the expressions R_{BP} and R_{NAT} model the bypass transition and the natural transition. The turbulent kinetic energy k_T is fed with energy (compare Equation A.1) as soon as transition is detected via

$$R_{\mathrm{BP}} = \frac{C_{R,\mathrm{BP}}\beta_{\mathrm{BP}}k_L\omega}{f_W} \quad \text{and} \quad R_{\mathrm{NAT}} = C_{R,\mathrm{NAT}}\beta_{\mathrm{NAT}}k_L\Omega. \tag{A.4}$$

Here, f_W represents a damping function that models wall damping effects, Ω is the magnitude of the mean rotation rate tensor and the constants $C_{R,\mathrm{BP}}$ and $C_{R,\mathrm{NAT}}$ are determined through model calibration.

The transition process itself is controlled by the threshold functions β_{BP} and β_{NAT} via

$$\beta_{\mathrm{BP}} = 1 - \exp\left(- \frac{\max\left[\left(\frac{k_T}{\nu\Omega} - C_{R,\mathrm{BP,crit}}\right), 0\right]}{A_{\mathrm{BP}}} \right). \tag{A.5}$$

A_{BP} is another model constant. All model constants used in the original settings are based on calibrations using a flat plate test and fully turbulent flow [106].

To verify the model implementation in OpenFOAM-1.6-ext, Klatt (2015) tests the k-k_L-ω model on a fully turbulent channel flow at a friction Reynolds number of $Re_\tau = 395$. The friction Reynolds number is based on the friction velocity u_τ, the channel half height h and the kinematic viscosity ν:

$$Re_\tau = \frac{u_\tau h}{\nu} = \frac{\sqrt{\frac{\tau_w}{\rho}}\, h}{\nu}. \tag{A.6}$$

Details on the case set-up are found in Klatt (2015). Results for comparison are available in form a model test [105] and DNS data [62].

First tests show that the implementation available in OpenFOAM 2.3.0 does not agree with the data found in the literature. A detailed description of the changes applied in the implementation can be found in Klatt (2015) and are also corrected in OpenFOAM 2.4.0. Results shown here all correspond to the corrected code version and can be seen in Figure A.1. Furthermore, the model results presented in the literature and the available DNS data are shown. The maximum deviation between the k-k_L-ω model and the DNS data reaches 5 %, which is considered a good agreement in the framework of RANS modelling and also agrees with the literature [105]. Although the magnitude of the maximum kinetic energy is under-predicted by 10 % in comparison with the DNS data, its position is correct (compare Figure A.4). As stated by Walters and Cokljat [105], the k-k_L-ω model is able to resolve the fully turbulent near-wall flow even better than other eddy-viscosity models. In a few sections some information are missing. This is caused by the poor resolution of the published data. The differences between the OpenFOAM 2.4.0 solution and the literature in the comparable sections are marginal.

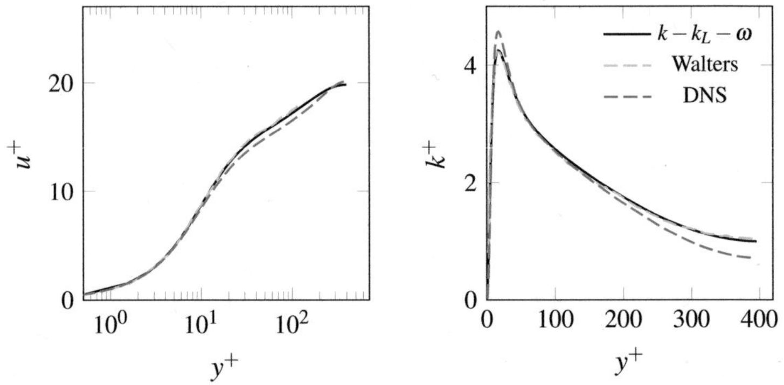

Figure A.4: Dimensionless (left) velocity and (right) turbulent kinetic energy profiles for a fully developed turbulent channel flow at $Re_\tau = 395$.

As already mentioned, the model constants R_{BP} and R_{NAT} feed the kinetic energy as soon as transition is detected. As such, the new calibration concentrates on the term R_{BP} as stated in Equation A.4. Klatt (2015) states that the model constant $C_{R,\text{BP}}$ is the most relevant coefficient if the effect strength of initiated bypass transition is to be calibrated. Changing this parameter from originally $C_{R,\text{BP}} = 0.12$ to $C_{R,\text{BP}} = 59$ results in a shift of the transitional Reynolds number in the presented pipe flow (compare Chapter 4.2) from 4600 to 3000.

A.4 Available Mitral Valve Models

The following table provides an overview over the research that was carried out on the MV. Only literature that takes the fluid flow into account is listed here. The overview is an extension of the literature summarised by Bakar (2015). Firstly, the sources are separated into the different available MV model types; i.e. diode type MV model (*diode*); planar MV model (*planar*); geometry-prescribed MV model (*geom.-pres.*); and fluid-structure interaction MV model (*FSI*). Secondly, the list is sorted alphabetically by the first authors' surname. Publications in a stationary framework are not included.

Completeness of the available literature is not guaranteed but the most impacting research is included to the best knowledge of the author. Because this work focuses on the modelling of the physiological MV, only a few examples that deal with prosthetic heart valves in the MV location are exemplary provided for additional reading.

Table A.1: Overview of MV models applied in the literature for CFD application.

	MV model type	**summary**
Le and Sotiropoulos [53]	diode	3D; IBM (CURVIB) framework; cell activation model determines LV movement; effect 3D valve is not expected to extend far from the MV tips
Lemmon and Yoganathan [54, 55]	diode	3D; IBM framework; LV and atrium incorporated by wound fibres; first description of atrial function; FSI between blood and tissue
Saber et al. [77]	diode	3D; ALE framework; combined MRI and CFD simulation; dominant flow features are qualitatively and quantitatively consistent with clinical experiments
Seo and Mittal [85] and Seo et al. [86]	diode	3D; IBM framework; model too simple to cover the complex fluid flow characteristics
Vedula et al. [102]	diode	3D; IBM framework; idealised LV; model matches well with experiment but also shows that matching with physiological conditions is challenging
Vierendeels et al. [104]	diode	2D; ALE framework; only filling flow is simulated

Watanabe et al. [109, 110]	diode	3D; ALE framework; FSI coupling between flow and ventricular wall; integrated sub-cellular molecular events
Baccani et al. [7]	planar	2D; axis symmetric; prescription through velocity profile at valve orifice; results include expected flow characteristics
Bavo et al. [8]	planar	3D; orifice projected from 3D valve; resulting vortex shape more regular and centred in comparison to 3D valve
Domenichini et al. [21]	planar	3D; ALE framework; shape of inlet jet prescribed; portion of a prolate spheroid
Krittian et al. [49]	planar	3D; ALE formulation; valve plane separated in idealised ring shapes; FSI between flow and ventricle wall
Nakamura et al. [65, 66]	planar	3D; examination of different valve opening modes; appearance of the vortex differs with the opening mode
Nordsletten et al. [67, 68]	planar	3D; orifice shape based on MRI data; flow profile prescribed; ALE formulation; FSI between flow and ventricle wall; valve model stable and effective
Schenkel et al. [80]	planar	3D; ALE framework; orifice shape based on MRI data; resulting fluid flow shows good agreement with the expected flow characteristics
Astorino et al. [5]	geom.-pres.	3D; no valve movement but two different states in diastole and systole; resistive IBM framework; efficient, flexible and robust

Bavo et al. [8]	geom.-pres.	3D; movement interpolated from segmented ultrasound images; ALE framework; recommendation for usage of 3D valve
Chnafa et al. [15]	geom.-pres.	3D; no valve movement but two different states in diastole and systole; LV moves in an ALE framework; simplifications valid if not oversimplified
Mihalef et al. [60]	geom.-pres.	3D; level-set framework; full heart model obtained from CT scans
Seo et al. [86]	geom.-pres.	3D; movement prescribed by varying leaflet angles over time; approach is found to be superior to a diode type MV model
Vedula et al. [103]	geom.-pres.	3D; movement prescribed by varying leaflet angles over time; inclusion of trabeculae and papillary muscles
Al-Atabi et al. [1]	FSI	2D; ALE framework; only diastolic phase with outflow through the apex; comparison with experiments show good agreement
Dahl et al. [17]	FSI	2D; rigid leaflets; ALE framework; results indicate that flow features might be missing if symmetric leaflets or an inadequate model for the left atrium are introduced
Espino et al. [24]	FSI	2D; valve remains closed; reaction on ventricular pressure during systole is evaluated; ALE framework
Kunzelman et al. [50]	FSI	3D; IBM framework; MV is surrounded by a computational box and not inserted into an LV

Stijnen et al. [94]	FSI	2D; rigid leaflets; IBM (fictitious domain) framework; with increasing St or Re, the functionality of the MV increases
Choi et al. [16]	prosthetic	3D; FSI within IBM framework; central hinge and implanted in anatomical orientation gives the best overall performance
Dumont et al. [22]	prosthetic	3D; ALE framework; St. Jude Regent Valve
Sotiropoulos and Borazjani [91]	prosthetic	review on CFD of bi-leaflet mechanical heart valves in aortic valve position; proper examination of the hinge regions remains challenging

A.5 Verification of the Porous Media Model

For validation of the porous media models a simple one-dimensional (1D) channel serves as test case. The bulk velocity at the channel inlet, u_b, and the pressure at the outlet, p_{out}, are prescribed. The resultant pressure drop over the channel length, Δp, is determined for comparison. An analytical solution is given by

$$\frac{\Delta p}{\rho} = \frac{p_{in}}{\rho} - \frac{p_{out}}{\rho}, \tag{A.7}$$

$$\frac{p_{in}}{\rho} = \frac{p_t}{\rho} - \frac{1}{2}u_b^2, \tag{A.8}$$

$$\frac{p_t}{\rho} = L u_b \left(\frac{\nu}{k_p} + \beta u_b \right) + \frac{p_{out}}{\rho}. \tag{A.9}$$

Quantitative values for the corresponding model constants are given in Table A.2.

$\nu\,[\mathrm{m^2\,s^{-1}}]$	$L\,[\mathrm{m}]$	$k_p\,[\mathrm{m^2}]$	$\beta\,[\mathrm{m^{-1}}]$	$\frac{p_{out}}{\rho}\,[\mathrm{m^2\,s^{-2}}]$
$3.8 \cdot 10^{-6}$	0.035	10^{-7}	2000	12.64

Table A.2: Model constants for the Darcy-Forchheimer porosity model.

For the numerical simulation a 3D-mesh has to be constructed. With only one cell in z-direction, a 2D-case is imitated. Symmetry boundary conditions at the upper and the lower wall of the channel enable a block velocity profile throughout the channel height and thus yield a 1D-profile. The initial condition of the flow field is set to u_b in x-direction and zero otherwise. Length and height are chosen as $L = 0.035\,\mathrm{m}$ and $H = 0.005\,\mathrm{m}$, respectively. Two pressure-velocity coupling algorithms are tested, the SIMPLE and the PIMPLE algorithm, in combination with the Darcy-Forchheimer porosity model and a steady mesh. Afterwards, the porosity model for moving meshes by

Wang et al. [107] is tested in combination with the PIMPLE method. Here, the upper and lower boundary are moving with u_b and thereby drive the flow. The mesh is moving with the walls.

Figure A.5 shows the resultant pressure gradient in the channel in dependency of the prescribed velocity. All simulations match the analytical solution perfectly.

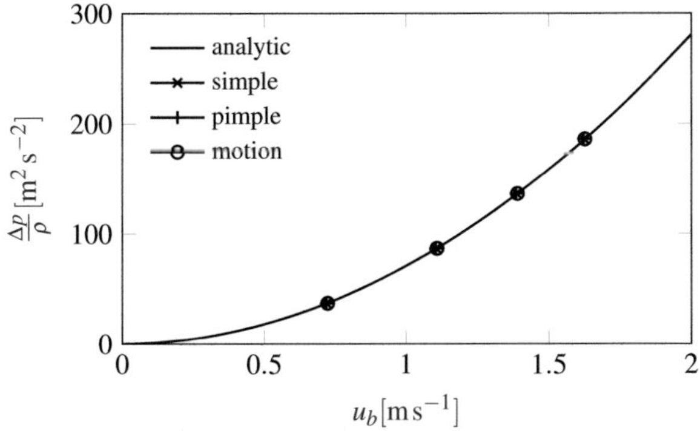

Figure A.5: Results of the porous 1D channel test case for different pressure-volume coupling algorithms and different porous media models.

Acknowledgements

As the final act of writing, I would like to take the opportunity to express my sincere thanks to everyone who has, directly or indirectly, contributed to this work.

First of all, I would like to thank my doctoral advisor, Prof. Dr.-Ing. Bettina Frohnapfel, for the opportunity to work under her guidance in the interesting field of biofluid mechanics. Thank you for your support and encouragement, the possibility to freely operate and take decisions and your firm trust in my skills. Further, I want to express my gratitude to Univ.-Prof. Dr.-Ing. habil. M. Breuer who not only agreed on being my second referee, but also supported my work with fruitful discussions, supplementary material and his expertise.

Many thanks to Prof. Dr. rer. nat. Olaf Dössel, Prof. Dr. Christian Wieners, Prof. Dr. Vincent Heuveline and their institute members who joined in the successful application at BMBF. My work is now part of the joint project "integriertes Herz-Modell", which fills me with pride. I also thank all students who conducted their theses under my guidance for their research contribution, their curiosity and their commitment. It is undeniable that I also learned a lot while (I tried) teaching you.

The impact of the working climate should not be underestimated. Thus, I deeply thank all current and former ISTM members for their long-term professional and moral support, for reading and letting read, for naivety when I borrow electronics and especially for their friendship. It's fun to travel with ISTM (!) and it has been a truly wonderful journey.

I thank my father and sister for taking the time to carefully read all these pages and my mother for cheering me up in the meantime. I love you. I also received continuous support from all my friends in the "Herde", who always help me figuring out my goals and clearing up my mind. Thank you!

As a matter of fact, I would not have written down all the lines without my husband who took a lot of the load off of me. Thank you so much, Ben, for your continuous encouragement, your honesty and your love. I love you to the moon and back and beyond. Besides, our wedding was the best wedding ever!